PLANNING HEALTH LESSONS:

Ideas for Effective Instruction

Wendy J. Schiff, M.S.

accompanies

Pollock/Middleton

SCHOOL HEALTH INSTRUCTION

●The Elementary & Middle School Years●

Third Edition

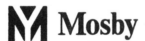 Mosby

Copyright © 1994 by Mosby-Year Book, Inc.
11830 Westline Industrial Drive
St. Louis, Missouri 63146

Printed in the United States of America

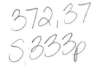

Preface

"Kids learn better by doing, not by sitting and having information pounded into their heads while they're not paying attention." These words were spoken by my 11 year-old, fifth-grader when asked what he thought of some of the activities that I prepared for this manual. His comments are very perceptive. Even college students find courses more enjoyable when the elements of exploration and discovery are woven into the educational setting. Lecture formats are "out;" *hands-on* guided discovery is "in."

Often student and novice teachers dread the task of developing lesson plans. It can be a time-consuming process. However with practice, experience, and creativity, lesson-planning becomes easier and more routine. Well-constructed lesson plans keep students engaged in the learning process and stimulated. Students who are busy learning new information and skills are easier to manage. Furthermore, administrators expect teachers to follow lesson plans that meet curriculum guidelines. Keep in mind there is no single, correct way to teach any content. Teachers have a repertoire of methodologies from which to design effective learning experiences. Age appropriateness, specific constraints of the classroom setting, and student learning characteristics play a role in choosing a method of presenting content or skills. Don't be afraid to "experiment" with a new idea to present information. You may want to discuss your idea with a veteran teacher or your mentor before trying it out on your class. When you do have an idea for an activity, ask yourself, "Does it meet my objectives? Does it maintain everyone's self-esteem? If it doesn't work, how can I change the activity so it is effective the next time?"

The purpose of this lesson planning guide is to provide student teachers with additional ideas for effective health education instruction. The following 120 lesson plans meet the student learning objectives listed on pages 83-86 of *School Health Instruction: The Elementary and Middle School*

Years, third edition by Marion Pollock and Kathleen Middleton. In addition to the lesson plans, the manual includes 40 student handouts and teacher resource ideas that support instruction.

Students majoring in education are aware that there are a variety of lesson-planning formats from which to choose. Certain formats are adopted by school districts and become "chiseled in stone." Other districts opt for more flexible methods; often, administrators are pleased if teachers prepare and teach from any well-designed lesson planning format. This manual uses a format that states the lesson's level (grades K through 8), title, content integration and generalization, and vocabulary. Each lesson lists the materials needed to conduct the activity, suggestions for initiating the activity ("anticipatory set"), the activity, and a form of closure. The materials identified as student handouts and teacher resources provide educational support for the activities. These include role-playing skits, patterns for designing bulletin boards and poster displays, answer keys to student handouts, and game instructions.

By using the lessons in this manual and those presented in the text, you have the foundation for effective health education. One of the major problems faced by elementary and middle-school teachers is finding the time to incorporate health content into a busy day. You will better serve the health educational needs of your students by taking the extra time to integrate health into other content areas. Health information becomes more real, more practical when it is integrated.

I would like to thank Jim Smith and Vicki Malinee, my editors at Mosby, for their enthusiastic support of my writing. Shannon Canty, Senior Production Editor, deserves acknowledgment for her careful and thorough review of this manual. The wonderful artwork for this project was produced by Donald O'Connor.

I wish you the best of luck as you prepare to be an educator of children!

Wendy Schiff, M.S.

TABLE OF CONTENTS

COMMUNITY HEALTH

TEACHING RESOURCES AND STUDENT HANDOUTS

PERSONAL HEALTH AND FITNESS
Student Objectives

Primary Level K-3 Student:

1.	Names health habits that protect self and others.
2.	Identifies physical, mental, and social benefits of good health.
3.	Explains why daily dental care is essential for the growth and development of sound teeth and gums.
4.	Describes ways decision making affects personal health practices.

Intermediate Level 4-5/6 Student:

1.	Explains ways personal health behavior is influenced by friends and family members.
2.	Describes the relationship of personal health behavior to the optimum structure and function of the body.
3.	Explains the relationship of physical fitness to sound body function.

Middle School Level 6/7-8 Student:

1.	Analyzes the relationship between diet choices and fitness.
2.	Designs personal health care and fitness programs to meet individual needs and interests.
3.	Describes both immediate and long-range effects of personal health care choices.

1

PERSONAL HEALTH AND FITNESS
PRIMARY LEVEL

Objective: Students should be able to name health habits that protect self and others.

Level: Kindergarten and grade 1

Title: *Brian, The Worm Collector*

Integration: Art, analysis skills

Vocabulary: Habits, germs

Content Generalization: Certain health habits promote health; others can lead to health problems and spread disease. Hands come in contact with bacteria and other organisms (germs) that spread disease. Simply washing dirty hands after using the bathroom is an important health habit to develop.

Materials: Bar of soap; jar; handout (Fig. 1-1) Brian, the Worm Collector; and crayons

Initiation: Place a bar of soap and a jar where students can see them.

Activity: Read the following story:

"Brian wanted to play outside one morning. He decided to dig in the garden and hunt for worms. Each time he found a wiggly worm, he placed it in his jar. When it was almost time for lunch, he heard his mother calling out, "Brian, Brian. Time to eat lunch!" He ran into the house with his jar of worms. He couldn't wait to show his mother the jar. Brian's mother was in the kitchen making sandwiches. What do you think she said when she saw Brian and his jar of worms?"

Children should be able to relate to this situation and suggest that his mother would want Brian to wash his hands before eating lunch. Ask children, "Why do we need to wash dirty hands with soap and warm water before eating?" Explain that germs are in dirt, and they can make people sick. Soap helps remove dirt. At this point, introduce the concept of **habits.** Ask children if they know what a habit is. Explain that habits are activities people do over and over again. Ask children if they have any habits that help keep them healthy such, as brushing their teeth. Ask children how they can make handwashing a habit.

Children can complete the picture by adding a worm, some dirt, and a jar to the picture before coloring it.

Closure: Ask, "Are there other times when people need to wash their hands?" Responses should include: before making food and after eating, going to the bathroom, coughing, and sneezing.

PERSONAL HEALTH AND FITNESS
PRIMARY LEVEL

Objective: Students should be able to identify physical, mental and social benefits of good health.

Level: Kindergarten through grade 3

Title: *I Am Healthy Because...*

Integration: Art, reading, analysis skills

Vocabulary: Healthy, habits

Content Generalization: Good health is the result of many factors including health habits and feelings about one's self and others. When one takes charge of their physical health, they feel good about themselves and others like to be around them.

Materials: Handout (Fig. 1-2) I Am Healthy Because..., crayons

Initiation: On the chalkboard, write " I am healthy because_____ "

Activity: Give children the handout. Read the partial statement that is written on the board and handout. Ask children to complete the sentence. (Kindergarten and first grade children will need your assistance to complete the statement on the handout.)

Children can finish the handout by drawing a picture of themselves involved in a health-promoting activity. Activities could include eating nutritious food, exercising, hugging a friend, or flossing their teeth.

Closure: When done, each child can display their artwork and read their statement to the rest of the class. Post their pictures on a bulletin board or outside of the classroom.

PERSONAL HEALTH AND FITNESS
PRIMARY LEVEL

Objective:	**Explain why daily dental care is essential for growth and development of sound teeth and gums.**
Level:	Grade 3
Title:	*Egg Shell Demonstration: The Battle Against Tooth Decay*
Integration:	Science, math, observational skills
Vocabulary:	Acid, corrosive, enamel, dentin, pulp, bacteria
Content Generalization:	The hardness of teeth is due to their mineral content, particularly the minerals calcium and phosphorus. Although very hard, tooth enamel can be destroyed by bacteria present in the mouth. These bacteria accumulate in a filmy layer called plaque on the surface of teeth. The bacteria release acid as a waste product. Acid damages the enamel layer and if untreated will destroy the inside parts of affected teeth. Frequent toothbrushing and flossing removedental plaque from teeth and help prevent tooth decay. Fluoride treatments strengthen teeth.
Materials:	6 hard-cooked eggs in shells, 32 oz. lemon juice, 1/2 cup measure, 6 small jars with lids, and tooth diagram poster (Fig. 1-3)
Initiation:	Place lemon juice and egg carton in a visible place.
Activity:	Divide class into six groups. Each group takes one egg and observes its shell's condition. Students should record this observation. Ask one student from each group to measure about 4 oz. of lemon juice and add it to the jar. Ask students about the nature of lemon juice. It is a food acid. What do they know about acids? Acids are corrosive, that is, they can destroy certain materials. Instruct students to place the egg into the lemon juice and allow one side to remain untouched by the juice. They should not disturb the jar for at least 4 hours. Later, have students take the egg out of the juice and examine the part of the shell that was in the juice and the part that was not exposed to the acid. They should record their observations and try to explain what occurred.

Using the poster, identify the structure of a tooth. Ask students if they can explain how bacteria can destroy the enamel and cause cavities to form. |
| **Closure:** | Ask, "How can you prevent cavities?" Children should mention the benefits of toothbrushing, flossing, using fluoride toothpastes, and visiting their dentist regularly. |

4

PERSONAL HEALTH AND FITNESS
PRIMARY LEVEL

Objective: Describes ways decision making affects personal health practices.

Level: Kindergarten and grade 1

Title: *Puppet Show: Derek's Busy Day*

Integration: Observation, prediction

Vocabulary: Decisions, choices, habits

Content Generalization: Decisions concerning health-related behaviors, such as hygienic practices, food choices, physical activity levels, and social interaction affect overall wellness.

Materials: Puppet stage, playground scene, kitchen scene, curtain to cover the table and hide puppeteer, script, dinosaur sock puppets, soap, toothbrush and toothpaste, apple, and candy bar

Initiation: Set up puppet show stage. Ask children to sit in front of the stage.

Activity: Derek the Dinosaur: " Hi kids! How are you today? (Pause) I 've learned a lot about health from my teacher, Mrs. T. Rex. I've learned so much about healthy choices, I'm not sure I can remember everything! Can you help me decide what to do today?" (Pause)

(A second dinosaur appears.) "Well, it's Derek! Do you want to play on the dino-bars or play tag?"

Derek: "Hi, Bernard, I don't know. I think I would rather watch TV or play my Game-dino video toy. Class, can you help me decide? (Pause) Why should I run around with Bernard?" Is exercise good for me?" (Pause)

"OK Bernard let's run around together!" (Puppets run around and play together.)

Derek: "Gee, Bernard, I am hungry now."

Bernard: "I have a candy bar we can share."

Derek: "I don't know if I should eat that, my mother gave me this apple." "Class, which should I choose?" (Pause, prepares to eat the apple.) "Oh, just look at my hands! They are so dirty!" What should I do? (Pause)

Bernard: "Yuk! Let's go into your house and wash them! **(Change of scene)**Bernard begins to wash hands at the sink, but he uses no soap.

Derek: "Wait Bernard, I think you are forgetting something.

Bernard: "Class, what am I forgetting to use?" (Pause) Oh, I forgot to use soap. This class is so smart!" "Derek, some of that candy stuck in my teeth, what should I do?"

Bernard: "I'm not sure, let's ask the class for help! Class, what can help Bernard clean the candy from his teeth? (Pause) Oh, of course, brush them!

5

(Derek picks up the toothbrush and with Bernard's help, places paste on it.)

Derek: "Wow, they are shiny now! I think we should go out and play again!

Bernard: "Great idea! You are my best friend. (Puppets hug.) "Let's go!"

Closure: Ask children if they can recall all of the good "dinosaur" health habits.

PERSONAL HEALTH AND FITNESS
INTERMEDIATE LEVEL

Objective:	**Explains ways personal health behavior is influenced by friends and family members.**
Level:	Grades 4 through 6
Title:	*Peer Pressure*
Integration:	Language arts, analysis
Vocabulary:	Peer pressure, influence, consequences
Content Generalization:	Personal health behaviors are influenced by many factors. At first, family members influence behavior. As children become older, the need for peer acceptance becomes a strong influence. Also, advertising exerts an influence on health-related decisions. Youngsters need to be able to recognize the impact of these influences (consequences) and determine when they are being pressured to make unwise choices.
Materials:	Prepare situation handouts with the five different situations described below.
Initiation:	Write "peer pressure" and "consequences" on the chalkboard. Ask students to try to define peer pressure and consequences.
Activity:	Divide students into groups. Give each group one of the situation handouts. Students are to analyze the situations, determine if peer pressure is involved, describe how the children in the situations may react, and recognize the consequences of each of the behavioral choices. The following are the situations:

1. Bobby has a friend, Kevin, who is in the seventh grade. When they are playing at Kevin's house, Kevin takes his father's gun out of a drawer. "Do you want to check this out?" Kevin asks.

2. While they are waiting for the bus, Deureka's friend, Sterling, offers her a cigarette. "This will help you lose weight," he says.

3. Takuji plays soccer with a group of friends. At one practice, they find a can of smokeless tobacco on the field. "Let's try this stuff!" says Kim.

4. Emory likes to ride his bike with Ted and Phil. One day Emory couldn't find his helmet. "That's OK." said Ted. "Emory looks stupid in that thing, anyway."

5. Maria and Elena are playing outside in the park when a teenage boy whom they do not know walks up to them and asks for help. "Will you help me find my lost puppy? he asks. "Oh, let's help him!" says Elena.

Ask each group to describe their situation and identify peer pressure influences, alternative behaviors, and consequences. Do the other students agree with each group's assessment of the situations?

Closure:	Ask students how they would handle similar pressure from peers.

PERSONAL HEALTH AND FITNESS
INTERMEDIATE LEVEL

Objective: **Describes the relationship of personal health behavior to the optimum structure and function of the body.**

Level: Grades 4 through 6

Title: *My Personal Health Log*

Integration: Language arts, analysis

Vocabulary: Logs

Content Generalization: Recording one's behavior and then analyzing the records to determine which habits can be altered is an important skill for anyone, including children. By eeping a journal of their health habits, children can use information gained in the classroom to analyze their behaviors and their health status.

Materials: Logs (small notebooks)

Initiation: Assign children to bring in a small notebook for the day of the activity.

Activity: Ask children to keep a log of their health habits for a week. Children are xpected to record each time they brush and floss their teeth, bathe, wash hands, eat breakfast, etc. Children will need to record when they go to sleep each night and at what time they wake up the next morning. They should also record how much time they spend watching TV and exercising. In addition to recording their actual behaviors, children should note how they felt each day.

At the end of the week's recording period, children should review their logs and write an essay explaining what they learned about their health habits. Did they make any changes in their normal routines because they were keeping the records? Are there any health habits that need to be changed? Did children notice any differences in the way they felt when they did not get enough sleep? Did they have trouble concentrating in school when they did not eat breakfast?

Closure: Do children report feeling better on the days when they exercised, ate breakfast, or had plenty of sleep? Is there a relationship between practicing good health habits and feeling better about yourself?

PERSONAL HEALTH AND FITNESS
INTERMEDIATE LEVEL

Objective:	**Explains the relationship of physical fitness to sound body functions.**
Level:	Grades 4 through 6
Integration:	Physical education, math, science
Title:	*Fitness and Heart Health*
Vocabulary:	Pulse, carotid artery
Content	
Generalization:	Being able to measure the pulse is an important safety and fitness skill. The carotid artery, which is along the side of the neck and under the lower jaw, is often easier for children to locate than the radial pulse in the wrist (Fig.1-4). The pulse represents the pressure in the artery when the blood is pumped out of the heart to the rest of the body. The resting pulse for 10 year-old children is around 70-110 beats per minute. Pulse rate increases with exercise since the heart has to pump more oxygen-rich blood to tissues for the release of energy. A person who is physically fit will have their pulse quickly return to normal after resting for a couple of minutes.
Materials:	Handout (Fig. 1-4) Locating Your Pulse
Initiation:	Have students move desks to clear an exercise area and pair up with nother student. Demonstrate how to find the carotid pulse.
Activity:	Have each child sit quietly and take their pulse for 15 seconds. Unless there s a clock with a second hand in the room, the teacher will need to keep time for the children. Ask students how they can estimate their pulse rate per minute by just measuring it for fifteen seconds (multiply 15 second value by 4 to obtain 60 second estimation). Students need to record this value.
	Explain that each member of the pair will perform jumping jacks for 1 minute. Children will be told when to begin jumping and when to stop. As soon as they stop jumping, they are to sit and take their pulse for 15 seconds. Again, they will be told when to stop counting. Each child should determine and record their exercise pulse rate per minute. Two minutes after the exercise has stopped, children who have jumped are to take their resting pulse and then determine and record the pulse rate per minute. Have the other member of the pair repeat the above activity and calculations.
	Ask students to evaluate the differences in pulse rates from the three measurements. Which children had the slowest exercise pulse rates? Which children had pulse rates that remained high 2 minutes after the jumping ceased? Which children believe they are very physically active?
Closure:	Ask, "Is there any relationship between the amount of physical activity you eceive and exercise pulse rate?" "How can your pulse rate be used to determine your state of physical fitness?"

PERSONAL HEALTH AND FITNESS
MIDDLE SCHOOL LEVEL

Objective: **Analyzes the relationship between diet choices and fitness.**

Level: Grades 6 through 8

Title: *Fats, Foods, and Fitness*

Integration: Science, math, physical education

Vocabulary: Calories, kcalories, grams

Content Generalization: A small amount of fat is essential in the diet, however, most Americans eat too much fat. Too much dietary fat can contribute to excess body fat, especially for people who do not get enough physical activity. If more Calories (kilocalories) are consumed than needed for energy, the excess is stored as body fat. (One pound of body fat represents about 3500 Calories.) Boys at this age need about 2500 Calories a day; girls need about 2200 Calories daily. Americans should consume no more than 30% of their total calories from fat. Children can learn to keep records of their food intake and stimate the total amount of calories contributed by fat.

Materials: Fat counter guides (food composition tables); if available, a computer program such as Mosby's ***Diet Simple*** and a computer for classroom use. Handouts: 3-day food record forms (see textbook, p. 324).

Activity: Ask children to keep 3-day food records. Children are to record everything they eat at mealtimes and snacks including sauces, condiments, and beverages. They need to try to estimate amounts in common measures such as cups and ounces. Information on food labels can help them determine some of the fat content of the food.

At the end of the recordkeeping period, have children determine how many Calories of fat they consumed each day. Each gram of fat supplies 9 Calories. Example: Sam determines that on one of his days he ate a total of 2700 Calories. He also ate 100 grams of fat. How many fat Calories did he consume? (Multiply 10 grams times 9 Calories/ gram = 900 Calories from fat.) To determine what percentage of his total day's intake was fat, take the number of Calories from fat (900) and divide it by the total number of Calories for the day (2700). He consumed one third of his Calories from fat.

Students then determine how long it would take Sam to gain one pound of fat if he ate 3200 Calories per day and did not increase his physical activity level. (He has increased his calorie intake by 500 Calories a day. Since 1 pound of body fat is approximately 3500 Calories, in 7 days he would have a surplus of 3500 Calories that would be stored as a pound of body fat.)

Closure: Ask, "If one wants to lose body fat, should they exercise more or eat less fat?"

PERSONAL HEALTH AND FITNESS
MIDDLE SCHOOL LEVEL

Objective: **Analyzes the relationship between diet choices and fitness.**

Level: Grades 6 through 8

Title: *More Fats, Foods, and Fitness*

Integration: Science, math

Vocabulary: Calories, kilocalories, grams

Content Generalization: A small amount of fat is essential in the diet, however, too much dietary fat can contribute to excess body fat, especially for people who do not get enough physical activity. Each pound of body fat represents 3500 Calories (kilocalories) of stored energy. The most effective way to lose body fat is to increase physical activity level and, if possible, reduce intake of excess Calories, especially from fatty snacks.

Materials: Food Calorie counter guides (food composition tables); if available, a computer program such as Mosby's *Diet Simple* and a computer for classroom use.

Handout (Fig. 1-5) Activities and Calories Burned Chart

Activity: Ask children to list five of their favorite foods. Have them analyze the caloric content of these foods using food composition tables or the computer program. Have children find activities they enjoy performing on the Activities and Calories Burned Chart. Ask students to estimate how much time it will take to burn up the kcalories consumed from their favorite foods list.

Closure: Why is just exercising not a very effective way to lose body fat?

Figure 1-5 is from Payne, Hahn: *Understanding Your Health*, 3/e, St. Louis, 1992, Mosby

11

PERSONAL HEALTH AND FITNESS
MIDDLE SCHOOL LEVEL

Objective:	**Designs personal health care and fitness program to meet individual needs and interests.**
Level:	Grades 6 through 8
Title:	*My Fitness Diary*
Integration:	Math, physical education
Content Generalization:	Youngsters can design a personalized physical fitness program and chart their progress.
Materials:	Handout (Fig. 1-6) Activity Graph
Initiation:	Prepare a poster-sized sample activity graph, and display it where it is visible. Invite a physical education teacher into the classroom to demonstrate proper and improper exercise techniques.
Activity:	Provide at least one graph handout for each student. Students are to choose at least three forms of physical activity to engage in for a minimum of 20 minutes a day. At the end of each activity period, students are to chart the amount of time (minutes) spent engaged in the activity and fill in the chart. The physical education teacher can assist by recording skinfold measurements on each student at the beginning of the recordkeeping period and again at the end. Changes in skinfolds indicate changes in body composition (i.e., a reduction in skinfold thickness represents a reduction in body fat stores).
Closure:	Ask students to explain the benefits of a personalized fitness plan.

PERSONAL HEALTH AND FITNESS
MIDDLE SCHOOL LEVEL

Objective: **Describes both immediate and long-range effects of personal health care choices.**

Level: Grades 7 and 8

Title: *Now and Then*

Integration: Language arts

Content Generalization: Health-care choices made at an early age influence health later in life. Negative health habits initiated in adolescence are often difficult to change.

Materials: Props for play

Initiation: Students are to "brainstorm" the components of a three-act play about negative and positive health-care choices that are made by young adolescents. The action should show the impact of these choices throughout life. For example, choosing to smoke cigarettes at age 14 can lead to lung disease later in life. Students are to create the characters, situations, and script. Each act should represent one of the stages of life.

Activity: Students take the story line created and develop the play. Some students can design the props, others can be a team of scriptwriters, and others, actors. Each student should have a "part" in the activity. This play can be staged for younger school-aged children.

Closure: Ask students to describe the immediate and long-range effects of the personal health-care choices that were presented in the play.

MENTAL AND EMOTIONAL HEALTH
Student Objectives

Primary Level K-3 Student:

1. Classifies social behaviors as acceptable and unacceptable.
2. Differentiates between pleasant and unpleasant emotions.
3. Illustrates ways to show friendship.

Intermediate Level 4-5/6 Student

1. Explains the difference between physical well-being and mental and emotional health.
2. Identifies positive and negative effects of stress.
3. Proposes acceptable ways to deal with strong negative emotions.

Middle School Level 6/7-8 Student

1. Identifies constructive ways to manage stress.
2. Analyzes the influence of peer pressure on health-related goals.
3. Describes the importance of setting realistic goals.
4. Explains the interrelationships among physical, mental, emotional. and social well-being.

MENTAL AND EMOTIONAL HEALTH
PRIMARY LEVEL

Objective:	**Classifies social behaviors as acceptable and unacceptable.**
Level:	Kindergarten through grade 2
Title:	*Mind Your Manners!*
Integration:	Language arts, comparisons
Vocabulary:	Manners
Content Generalization:	Manners are valuable for social acceptance.
Materials:	Obtain a copy of *Hello, Gnu. How Do You Do?* by Barbara Shook Hazen, Doubleday, NY, 1990 (ISBN: 0-385-26449-6)
Initiation:	Write "Manners" on the board. Have children sit on floor in preparation for storytelling. Ask children to define manners.
Activity:	Read sections of the book and show illustrations to children. After each situation presented in the book, ask children to describe what the animals did that showed good or bad manners.
Closure:	Ask children to give examples of good and bad manners.

MENTAL AND EMOTIONAL HEALTH
PRIMARY LEVEL

Objective: **Differentiates between pleasant and unpleasant emotions.**

Level: Kindergarten and grade 1

Title: *Sad Day, Happy Day*

Integration: Language arts, art

Vocabulary: Emotions

Content Generalization: Emotions are an important component of human behavior. Children need to be able to differentiate between how they feel when they are sad or happy. Recognizing these feelings will help make them feel more comfortable with themselves and others.

Materials: Handout (Fig. 2-1) Sad Day, Happy Day

Initiation: At first, the teacher makes a sad face and asks children to describe how the teacher feels. Then the teacher makes a happy face and asks students to describe how the teacher feels. Ask children to make happy and sad faces.

Activity: Give children the handout, and ask them to draw a picture of themselves doing something that makes them happy and another one of something that makes them sad.

Closure: Ask children what they can do to make themselves feel happy when they feel sad.

MENTAL AND EMOTIONAL HEALTH
PRIMARY LEVEL

Objective:	**Illustrate ways to show friendship.**
Level:	Kindergarten and grade 1
Title:	*Friends are Special People*
Integration:	Reading readiness, art, analysis
Vocabulary:	Friends, friendship
Content Generalization:	Establishing and maintaining friendships are important components of emotionally healthy behavior. Friends are people who enjoy being together, sharing experiences, and expressing feelings. Friends care about each other.
Materials:	Sheets of paper, crayons
Initiation:	Write the words "friends" and "friendship" on the board. Ask children to "brainstorm" the following question, "What do you think of when you hear the word friends?" "Why do we need friends?" "What does a person do to make friends?"
Activity:	Ask children to draw a picture of themselves doing something fun with one or more of their friends.
Closure:	Ask, "How do we show someone that we want to be their friend?"

MENTAL AND EMOTIONAL HEALTH
INTERMEDIATE LEVEL

Objective: **Explains the difference between physical well-being and mental and emotional health.**

Level: Grades 4 and 5

Title: *My Mentalmeter*

Integration: Language arts

Vocabulary: Physical health, mental and emotional health

Content Generalization: The concept of physical health is less abstract than mental and emotional health. For example, one can see a rash, record the temperature of a fever, or view an x-ray film of a broken bone. Measuring mental and emotional health is more difficult because people often hide their real feelings.

Materials: Handout (Fig. 2-2) Mentalmeter

Initiation: Display a poster of the "mentalmeter". Write "physical health" and "mental/emotional health" on the board. Divide the class into teams of four or five students. Give each team about 5-10 minutes to come up with definitions of mental/emotional health and physical health. Students should be able to give examples of people who are emotionally as well as physically healthy.

Activity: Give each student a copy of the mentalmeter handout. Ask each students to construct a mentalmeter. The mentalmeter shows the intensity of their emotions as they perceive them during various situations. Students are to label points on the meter that represent relaxed mental states and identify situations in which they would be relaxed. After identifying the relaxed states, students need to label points on the meter that indicate where they would obtain a measurement as they become increasingly upset. They need to describe the situations that cause that level of emotional discomfort. Finally, they need to identify situations in which they are extremely upset and label that point on the meter.

Closure: Ask, "What can you do to reduce the level of your mentalmeter?"

18

MENTAL AND EMOTIONAL HEALTH
INTERMEDIATE LEVEL

Objective: **Identifies positive and negative effects of stress.**

Level: Grades 4 through 6

Title: *The Day My Rubber Band Almost Broke!*

Integration: Language arts

Vocabulary: Stress, stress management

Content Generalization: Stress is a part of living. Learning to manage stress in positive ways is crucial for optimal physical and mental and emotional health. Positive ways of dealing with stress include engaging in hobbies, talking to a trusted friend, or exercising. Negative ways of dealing with stress include fighting, saying hurtful things to others, engaging in reckless behavior, or abusing drugs.

Materials: Small journals, large rubber band

Initiation: Teacher stretches rubber band while describing how stress can make people feel "stretched to the limit".

Activity: Ask students to recall a day in which they felt "stretched" to their limit. Have them write a story about that day's incidents.

Closure: Ask, "Did you handle the stressful situation in a negative or positive manner?"

MENTAL AND EMOTIONAL HEALTH
INTERMEDIATE LEVEL

Objective: **Proposes acceptable ways to deal with strong negative emotions.**

Title: *Conflict Control Contracts*

Level: Grades 4 through 6

Integration: Language arts, social studies

Vocabulary: Conflicts, resolution

Content Generalization: Youngsters need to learn ways to resolve disagreements without physically or emotionally injuring others. Agreeing to resolve conflicts while maintaining human dignity is possible by establishing behavioral contracts.

Materials: None

Initiation: Ask students to give an example of a conflict that has occurred in current national or international events. Ask students how these conflicts are resolved. Are the outcomes positive or negative?

Activity: Discuss situations involving student conflicts that have occurred in school or on the bus. What factors contributed to the conflict? How were they resolved?

Ask students to design a contract in which each student will agree to resolve disagreements in a positive rather than negative manner. After students sign the contracts, display them on the bulletin board.

Closure: If disagreements occur that are similar to the ones described earlier, how will the individuals involved resolve them in a positive manner?

MENTAL AND EMOTIONAL HEALTH
INTERMEDIATE LEVEL

Objective:	**Proposes acceptable ways to deal with strong negative emotions.**
Level:	Grades 7 and 8
Title:	*Conflict Court*
Integration:	Language arts, social studies
Vocabulary:	Retribution
Content Generalization:	Youngsters need to learn ways to resolve disagreements without physically or emotionally injuring others. The court system is important in societies as a means of resolving conflicts.
Materials:	Gavel prop
Initiation:	Invite a lawyer into class to describe how conflicts are resolved in civil courts.
	This activity can culminate the in study of the judicial system.
Activity:	Students fabricate the situation that leads to a disagreement occurring between two students.
	A student "jury" is selected from the class. Two students are to play the part of the individuals involved in the conflict. Both present their case to the jury.
	The jury decides the outcome of the conflict and recommends some form of retribution.
Closure:	Ask students how personal disagreements can be resolved in a similar fashion.
	Do they wish to establish a classroom "court" to air disagreements?

MENTAL AND EMOTIONAL HEALTH
MIDDLE SCHOOL LEVEL

Objective: **Identifies constructive ways to manage stress.**

Level: Grades 6 through 8

Title: *Blow-out Time*

Integration: Music

Vocabulary: None

Content
Generalization: Deep breathing is a simple, quick, and effective way to relax.

Materials: Tape cassette of ocean waves, gentle rain, or slow music. Tape player

Initiation: Begin playing tape softly. Turn off artificial lights, and allow natural light into the room.

Activity: While listening to the tape player, have children practice taking in deep breaths, then exhaling. After about six repetitions, ask students how they feel.

Closure: Ask, "When do you think it would be a good time to practice deep breathing?"

The idea is for them to connect deep-breathing exercises with relaxing before or during stressful situations.

MENTAL AND EMOTIONAL HEALTH
MIDDLE SCHOOL LEVEL

Objective:	**Analyzes the influence of peer pressure on health related choices.**
Title:	*Peer Power*
Integration:	Language arts
Vocabulary:	Positive peer pressure, negative peer pressure
Content Generalization:	Peer pressure influences decisions youngsters make concerning health choices. Important skills include being able to recognize when peer pressure occurs and analyze the situation to avoid negative outcomes.
Materials:	Handout (Fig. 2-3) Peer Power
Initiation:	Ask for six volunteers (three boys and three girls). Pair volunteers into three teams: 1) two boys, 2) two girls, and 3) a boy and a girl. Give each team the appropriate handout. Teams will need about 5 minutes to review their role-play situation and prepare for the activity. While they are in preparation, ask the class to brainstorm to think of situations involving positive and negative peer pressure.
Activity:	Have each team act out their role-play situation for the rest of the class. After each pair role plays, ask students to decide if the situation involved positive or negative peer pressure.
Closure:	How can you decide if a situation involves negative or positive peer pressure?

MENTAL AND EMOTIONAL HEALTH
MIDDLE SCHOOL LEVEL

Objective:	**Describe the importance of setting realistic goals.**
Level:	Grades 7 and 8
Title:	*Exploring My Future*
Integration:	Language arts, interpersonal skills
Vocabulary:	Occupations, aptitude
Content Generalization:	Adolescence is the time to be thinking about the future. By investigating occupations, youngsters can determine what steps need to be taken while they are still in school to prepare for the future.
Materials:	None
Initiation:	Invite the high school guidance counselor into class to discuss ways to determine if interests and aptitude can be used for career selection. The counselor can explain how courses taken at the high school level can prepare one for a particular vocation or college.
Activity:	Have students select an occupation that interests them. Ask them to investigate what educational steps are necessary to prepare for that career. They need to identify someone working in that field and interview him or her about their job. What do they like most about it? What aspects of the job are unpleasant?
	Students will be asked to write a report of their career exploration and give a brief report to the class.
Closure:	Ask students, "What can you do now to prepare for a future career?"

MENTAL AND EMOTIONAL HEALTH
MIDDLE SCHOOL LEVEL

Objective:	**Explains the relationships among physical, mental, and emotional, and social well being.**
Level:	Grades 7 and 8
Title:	*The Wellness Puzzle*
Integration:	Science, language arts
Vocabulary:	None
Content Generalization:	Physical, mental and emotional, and social health are all interrelated. When there is a decline in any one of these wellness components, the others are negatively affected.
Materials:	Three cards: (1) physical health, (2) mental and emotional health, and (3) social health.
Initiation:	Divide the class into three groups. Give each group a card. Separate the chalkboard into thirds. In each third, write at the top of each section physical health, mental and emotional health and social health.
either:	
Activity:	Ask students in each group to brainstorm examples of their wellness component. For example, the physical health group could identify eating a nutritious diet and getting enough sleep. After about 5 minutes, have them write their list on the board in the appropriate section. Ask students what they believe can happen if one of these components becomes less healthy, for example, if they don't get enough sleep. How does that affect their school work? Their social life?
Closure:	Ask students to write an essay describing how their physical condition affects their mental and emotional as well as social conditions.

FAMILY LIFE
Student Objectives

Primary Level K-3 Student:

1. Defines the meaning of family.
2. Identifies responsibilities and privileges of various family members.
3. Describes ways family membership changes.
4. Explains that all living things come from other living things.

Intermediate Level 4-5/6 Student:

1. Proposes constructive ways to solve conflicts with friends and family.
2. Interprets changes in social activities as family members change.
3. Describes the progression of the individual through the life cycle from birth to death.
4. Identifies growth and developmental characteristics common in puberty.

Middle School Level 6/7-8 Student:

1. Predicts physical, mental and emotional, and social changes that occur during adolescence.
2. Explains why growth and development is individual, although predictable.
3. Describes the reproductive processes.
4. Identifies social and cultural factors in the development of responsible health behavior.

FAMILY LIFE
PRIMARY LEVEL

Objective:	**Defines the meaning of family.**
Level:	Kindergarten
Title:	*Our Family Tree*
Integration:	Art
Vocabulary:	Families
Content Generalization:	Most families are made up of people related to each other, such as parents and their children. Families may not have both parents living in the household. Many families are made up of different families, such as when divorced people with children marry. However, family members often stay together because they care about and want to help each other.
Materials:	Our Family Tree bulletin board (Fig. 3-1)
Initiation:	Prepare bulletin board.
Activity:	Have children draw a picture of their family, identifying the members for the bulletin board display. Children can help arrange the pictures on the bulletin board.
Closure:	Ask, "What makes your family special?"

FAMILY LIFE
PRIMARY LEVEL

Objective: **Identifies responsibilities and privileges of various family members.**

Level: Grades 1 and 2

Title: *Class Menagerie*

Integration: Language arts, comparisons

Vocabulary: Responsibilities, chores

Content Generalization: Each family member has a role to play in supporting the family. This helps divide up the household responsibilities and teaches the benefits of cooperation.

Materials: Chore Chart (Fig 3-2), Gold sticker stars

Initiation: Ask the class to help the teacher make a list of all of the jobs that are necessary to keep the classroom running smoothly. Their ideas can be used to complete the chore chart.

Activity: Ask children to choose a responsibility to be carried out within a given time period. Explain that children are to read the chore chart at the beginning of each day to find out what they are expected to do. Rotate chores every week so that each child will have a new responsibility. Place a gold star next to each child's name on the chart after they carry out their chore for the week.

Closure: Ask children to compare the classroom with its chores to their family life at home. What kinds of chores to they have at home? Why should they help at home?

FAMILY LIFE
PRIMARY LEVEL

Objective:	**Describes ways family membership changes.**
Level:	Kindergarten and grade 1
Title:	*My Family Has Changed*
Integration:	Observation and description
Vocabulary:	Families, adopt
Content Generalization:	Family membership changes for many reasons. Some are sad reasons, such as the death of a parent or grandparent. Other reasons are happy occasions, such as when a baby brother or sister is born. Change is a part of life.
Materials:	The book, *All Kinds of Families*, by Norma Simon, Chicago, 1976, Albert Whitman & Co. (ISBN: 0-8075-0282-0)
Initiation:	Ask children to prepare for "storytelling time."
Activity:	Read *All Kinds of Families* to children.
Closure:	Ask, "Let's think of all of the reasons why families change."

FAMILY LIFE
PRIMARY LEVEL

Objective:	**Explains that all living creatures come from other living things.**
Level:	Kindergarten through grade 2
Title:	*Animal Parents, Animal Babies*
Integration:	Science, observation
Vocabulary:	None
Content Generalization:	Living things produce similar living things. Small animals in the classroom provide opportunities for teaching responsibilities and show that animals can produce babies.
Materials:	Aquarium, guppies, and supplies. Male and female hamsters, gerbils or other small rodents; cages, and supplies
Initiation:	Set up an area in the classroom for keeping animals. Ask children to volunteer to help take care of the animals. Have a contest to name the animals. Ask if any children have pets. Did their pets ever have babies? What did the babies look like?
Activity:	Have children count the number of fish in the aquarium and describe their size. When any baby fish are discovered, have the children compare them to the parents. Children are also likely to observe the birth of baby rodents. Ask children to compare the appearance of the baby rodents at birth to those of the baby fish. How are they similar; how are they different?
Closure:	Ask, "Where do baby fish come from?" "Where do baby hamsters come from?"

FAMILY LIFE
INTERMEDIATE LEVEL

Objective: **Proposes constructive ways to solve conflicts with friends and family.**

Level: Grades 4 through 6

Title: *Act Right, Don't Fight*

Integration: Language arts, problem solving

Vocabulary: Conflict resolution

Content Generalization: Conflicts arise between family members and friends in everyday life. To maintain harmony, conflict resolution skills that avoid harming others must be practiced. Positive conflict resolution involves finding solutions that do not hurt others and preserve relationships.

Initiation: Ask how many students had a disagreement with a friend or family member that resulted in losing the friend or straining the family relationship.

Activity: Ask students to write an essay about the incident and how they could have resolved it without losing their friend or straining their relationship with family.

Closure: Ask, "Why are conflict resolution techniques that preserve feelings important when you're are working out differences with others?"

FAMILY LIFE
INTERMEDIATE LEVEL

Objective:	**Interprets changes in social activities as family members mature.**
Level:	Grades 5 and 6
Title:	*Please, I'm Not a Kid Anymore*
Integration:	Language arts, analysis
Vocabulary:	Maturation, siblings
Content Generalization:	As family members mature, social expectations change. This often creates conflicts within families. Youngsters can recognize differences in the treatment given to members of the family and explore reasons why those differences occur. Increasing responsibilities, such as helping out or paying for material items, are ways parents prepare children to function on their own.
Initiation:	Write the words "maturation" and "siblings" on the chalkboard. Ask students to define these terms. Ask how many students have older brothers or sisters. Ask if they notice differences in the way they are treated compared to themselves. How many have younger siblings? Does maturation of family members involve changes in your parents' expectations?
Activity:	Ask students to write an essay about the ways members of their family are treated differently.
Closure:	Ask students why do they think there are differences in the way family members are treated. What role does maturity have in this process of change?

FAMILY LIFE
INTERMEDIATE LEVEL

Objective:	**Describes the progression of the individual through the life cycle from birth to death.**
Level:	Grade 4
Title:	*Memories*
Integration:	Social studies, art, interpersonal
Vocabulary:	None
Content Generalization:	Aging begins from the moment life begins. The life span consists of predictable stages as one passes from infancy to old age.
Materials:	Invitations
Initiation:	Explain that a panel discussion with aging adults will form the focus of a lesson on the life span. Have students identify eight people past the age of 65. Students design and prepare letters to invite these individuals to participate in the panel discussion. Students prepare questions to ask visitors about what it is like to be an older adult.
Activity:	Arrange visitors' seating in the center of the classroom; students arrange their desks in a semi-circle around the guests. As the guests to spend about one-half hour discussing what life was life when they were the students' age.
Closure:	Have students write thank you notes to the visitors expressing what they learned about aging.

FAMILY LIFE
INTERMEDIATE LEVEL

Objective: **Describes the progression of the individual through the life cycle from birth to death.**

Level: Grade 4

Title: *Baby, Look At You Now!*

Integration: Social studies, art, interpersonal

Vocabulary: Adolescence

Content Generalization: Aging begins from the moment life begins. The life span consists of predictable stages as one passes from infancy to old age. Adolescents retain many features that were apparent when they were infants.

Materials: Baby photos, "Baby Look At You Now!" bulletin board.

Initiation: Ask students to bring in a baby picture, preferably one in which they are less than 2 years old. Tell them not to show the picture to others in the class. Explain that the picture will be tacked up on the bulletin board; they should check with their parents to make sure this is OK. The teacher should include one of his or her baby photos.

Activity: The teacher collects the photos and places them on the classroom bulletin board. Students try to identify which student is in each baby photo. They write their guesses next to the photo. After a day, the students reveal their baby photo identity.

Closure: Ask students to identify the most obvious changes that occur as they pass from early childhood into adolescence.

FAMILY LIFE
INTERMEDIATE LEVEL

Objective:	**Identifies growth and developmental characteristics common in puberty.**
Level:	Grades 5 and 6
Title:	*My Diary of Changes*
Integration:	Science, language arts
Vocabulary:	Puberty
Content Generalization:	As boys and girls enter puberty, they need to be aware that many physical and emotional changes are normal at this time of life. Their increasing levels of sex hormones are responsible for the physical changes, as well as the emotional ones. Puberty begins with the first signs of reproductive organ maturation, generally around ages 9-11 for girls and 11-13 for boys.
Materials:	Personal logs or diaries
Initiation:	Give logs to students. Write "puberty" on the chalkboard. Ask students to define the term. Invite the school nurse into the classroom to answer youngsters' questions about physical and emotional changes associated with puberty.
Activity:	Students are to keep a personal diary of their physical and emotional changes experienced at this time. This diary should not be identified with their names. The teacher may ask to collect the diaries from time to time, but anonymity is important. Announce that if youngsters are having any troublesome problems, they should talk to the school nurse or guidance counselor.
Closure:	Ask students to brainstorm and list the physical and emotional changes that occur with puberty.

FAMILY LIFE
MIDDLE SCHOOL LEVEL

Objective:	**Predicts physical, mental and emotional, and social changes that occur during adolescence.**
Level:	Grades 6 through 8
Title:	*What's Happening To Me!*
Integration:	Language arts, interpersonal
Vocabulary:	Adolescence, puberty
Content Generalization:	As boys and girls enter puberty, they need to be aware that many physical and emotional changes are normal at this time of life. Their increasing levels of sex hormones are responsible for the physical changes, as well as the emotional ones. Puberty begins with the first signs of reproductive organ maturation, generally around ages 9-11 for girls and 11-13 for boys. These changes can have positive or negative impacts on social relationships. Communication with parents is extremely important at this time.
Materials:	Male and female body patterns poster (Fig. 3-3)
Initiation:	Place poster where students can see it. Ask student to identify the obvious, physical (visible) changes the bodies go through during puberty and emotional and social changes that are not so obvious. List changes on the board.
Activity:	Have students talk to their parents to find out how old they were when they went through puberty and if they can recall how it affected them emotionally and socially. Students are to write an essay comparing their parents' experience to theirs.

FAMILY LIFE
MIDDLE SCHOOL LEVEL

Objective: **Explains why growth and development is individual, although predictable.**

Level: Grades 6 through 8

Title: *Of Peanuts and People*

Integration: Science, math, observation

Vocabulary: Variation, heredity, species, frequency

Content Generalization: Variation (individual differences) occurs in all living things, even in the same species. Although all humans are members of the same species and look similar, each is different. One of the differences that varies is maturation. Living things mature at different rates. This is explained by heredity, genetic information that dictates an individual's unique characteristics. Genetic information is passed from one generation to the next. One of the inherited characteristics is maturity rate. Some mature earlier than others. Recording the frequency of some human characteristic provides students with concrete information about normal variation.

Materials: A bag of peanuts in shells, rulers, measuring tape, masking tape

Initiation: Students are to team up with a partner. Each team takes about five peanuts. Ask them to examine the peanuts and record how each is similar and different. Place a long strip of masking tape on far side of the chalkboard. Using the measuring tape, record measures on the masking tape from 4 feet 6 inches through 5 feet 10 inches. Indicate half-inch intervals along the masking tape.

Activity: Ask students to take turns measuring and recording each other's height, using the masking tape measuring guide. One person from each team writes both of their heights on the chalkboard. When everyone's height is listed, have students place the different heights in order from shortest to tallest. In some cases, more than one individual will be the same height. To show the frequency of each measurement, place the number of individuals who are that height next to the measurement.

Closure: Ask students why there are differences in peanuts and their heights. What role does heredity play in determining an individual's maturation rate?

FAMILY LIFE
MIDDLE SCHOOL LEVEL

Objective:	**Describes the reproductive processes.**
Level:	Grades 7 and 8
Title:	*Miracle of Life*
Integration:	Science
Vocabulary:	Conception, fertilization, embryo, embryonic, fetus, fetal

Content Generalization: Human reproduction involves the union of a sperm cell from a male and an egg from a female. This is called fertilization or conception. The fertilized egg becomes attached to the inside of the female's uterus, where it goes through embryonic and fetal stages before birth.

Materials: Video: *The Miracle of Life*, produced by Sveriges Television in association with WGBH Boston. Available from Crown Video, New York, NY, (212) 254-1600. Blank paper or notecards for questions.

Initiation: A week before showing the video, hand out a parent approval letter similar to the one shown on p. 305 in the text. Give students a date to return the signed letter. Give students paper or notecards for questions. Make certain that students have returned the parental approval form. Students who have not returned the form should be assigned the task of talking to their parents about human reproduction as an educational alternative. Arrange to have the school library manage those students while those who have obtained parental permission view the video.

Activity: Show the video. After the video, ask students to write any questions about human reproduction on the paper or notecard and turn them in. Read their questions and ask the students to try to answer them.

Closure: Ask students to describe the steps a human egg and sperm must go through before a baby is born.

FAMILY LIFE
MIDDLE SCHOOL LEVEL

Objective:	**Describes the reproductive processes.**
Level:	Grades 7 and 8
Title:	*The Miracle of Life: The Play*
Integration:	Science, language arts
Vocabulary:	Sexual intercourse, conception, fertilization, embryo, embryonic, fetus, fetal
Content Generalization:	Human reproduction involves the union of a sperm cell from a male and an egg from a female. Sperm are produced in the male testes, and eggs mature in the female ovaries. During sexual intercourse, sperm are released into the female's reproductive tract. If one sperm enters an egg, fertilization or conception has occurred. The fertilized egg becomes attached to the inside of the female's uterus, where it goes through embryonic and fetal stages before birth.
Materials:	Plain cardboard for signs, marking pen, yarn
Initiation:	Before this activity, all students need to have returned the parental approval form (a sample is shown on p. 305 of the text). An alternative project should be assigned to those students who have not returned the form.
Activity:	Have students volunteer to work in play production teams. The largest team will write the script for a play about human reproduction. This team needs to list all of the characters, such as the organs involved, "egg," and "sperm cells." The second team makes the signs to identify the characters. The signs will need to have two holes punched into them and be made into "necklaces" using the yarn. Actors wear these for identification. The last team directs the play. After a reasonable period of time for production and rehearsals, have students act out the human reproductive process from sperm and egg cell to birth.
Closure:	Ask students to write a paragraph describing the human reproductive process.

FAMILY LIFE
MIDDLE SCHOOL LEVEL

Objective: Identifies social and cultural factors in the development of responsible health behaviors.

Level: Grades 6 through 8

Title: *Sex Can Wait*

Integration: Social studies, language arts, analysis

Vocabulary: Sexual intercourse, abstinence, abstention

Content Generalization: In our society, children need to have a great deal of preparation for their adult roles. Although they are physically capable to become parents during early adolescence, they are not emotionally or financially ready for this major responsibility. Youngsters need to recognize the consequences of premature parenthood on themselves, their families and society. Therefore they need to abstain from sexual intercourse until they are prepared to handle the responsibilities of parenthood.

Materials: Information about current teenage pregnancy rates and the consequences of teen pregnancy available from Planned Parenthood.

Initiation: Before this activity, all students need to have returned the parental approval form (a sample is shown on p. 305 of the text). An alternative project should be assigned to those students who have not returned the form. Write "teen pregnancy" on the chalkboard. Ask them to identify the physical, emotional, and social problems associated with teen pregnancy. Why is it a national problem?

Activity: Write "sexual intercourse" and "abstinence" on the chalkboard. Ask them to define these terms. Ask students to determine when is the best age to become a parent. What factors need to be considered before engaging in sexual intercourse? Are they prepared to become parents at this time?

Closure: Ask each student to write a paragraph that identifies the physical, emotional, and social reasons why he or she should abstain from sexual intercourse.

NUTRITION
Student Objectives

Primary Level K-3 Student:

1. Lists distinctive characteristics of foods.
2. Explains the importance of eating a variety of foods.
3. Describes food combinations that provide a balanced diet.
4. Identifies snack foods that are nutritious.

Intermediate Level 4-5/6 Student:

1. Indentifies factors that influence personal food choices.
2. Classifies foods according to their major nutrients.
3. Analyzes the nutritional value of food choices for meals and snacks.
4. Explains reasons for different nutritional requirements between individuals.

Middle School Level 6/7-8 Student:

1. Evaluates diets appropriate for individual needs.
2. Explains the relationship between caloric intake, level of activity, and body weight.
3. Analyzes nutritional value of food in fad diets.
4. Predicts long-range outcomes of poor diet choices.

NUTRITION
PRIMARY LEVEL

Objective: **Lists distinctive characteristics of foods.**

Level: Kindergarten

Title: *Tongues Are for Tasting*

Integration: Reading readiness, description, art

Vocabulary: Sour, sweet, salty, spicy, tart, bitter, fatty

Content Generalization: Children learn to recognize foods by characteristics, including appearance, feel, and taste. This prepares them for recognizing nutritional differences, such as foods that are high in fat, salt, or sugar. Foods that taste good are not necessarily the most nutritious.

Materials: Paper, crayons

Initiation: Ask children to brainstorm words to describe how foods taste. Write these words on the chalkboard.

Activity: Ask children to identify a food that tastes sweet, salty, sour, bitter, or fatty.

Closure: Ask children to draw a picture of their favorite food and copy the word from the board that matches how it tastes.

NUTRITION
PRIMARY LEVEL

Objective: **Explains the importance of eating a variety of foods.**

Level: Grade 3

Title: *Search for the Perfect Food*

Integration: Science

Vocabulary: Nutrients

Content Generalization: Foods are mixtures of nutrients. No single food that occurs in nature is complete, that is, contains all of the nutrients needed to support life. Therefore we need to eat a variety of foods from all of the major food categories shown in the Food Pyramid for good health.

Materials: Food composition tables

Initiation: Ask students to list the characteristics of a perfect food. Write their suggestions on the chalkboard.

Activity: Ask students to identify a naturally occurring food that they think is "perfect." Have them look up the food in the food composition tables to see if it contains all of the major nutrients.

Closure: Ask students, "Since no single natural food contains all of the nutrients needed, how can you be sure that your diet is nutritious?"

NUTRITION
PRIMARY LEVEL

Objective:	**Explains the importance of eating a variety of foods.**
Level:	Kindergarten
Title:	*Pyramid Puzzle*
Integration:	Reading readiness
Vocabulary:	Nutrients, pyramid
Content Generalization:	Foods are mixtures of nutrients. No single food that occurs in nature is complete, that is, contains all of the nutrients needed to support life. Therefore we need to eat a variety of foods from all of the major food categories shown in the Food Pyramid for good health.
Materials:	Six Food Pyramid puzzles made by using heavy cardboard. Copy the puzzle parts as shown in Fig. 4-1. Laminate to protect puzzle pieces. Store puzzle pieces in an envelope.
Initiation:	Explain that no single food contains all of the nutrients needed for living. Nutrients are the materials found in food that help us grow, learn, and play. People need to eat many different foods to stay healthy. Divide the class into cooperative groups, each consisting of three or four children.
Activity:	Give each group an envelope with the pyramid puzzle. Have them put it together. Check their puzzles.
Closure:	Ask why it is important to eat food from all six pieces of the puzzle?

NUTRITION
PRIMARY LEVEL

Objective:	**Explains the importance of eating a variety of foods.**
Level:	Grade 1
Title:	*Pyramid Bulletin Board*
Integration:	Reading readiness, art
Vocabulary:	Nutrients, pyramid
Content Generalization:	Foods are mixtures of nutrients. No single food that occurs in nature is complete, that is, contains all of the nutrients needed to support life. Therefore we need to eat a variety of foods from all of the major food categories shown in the Food Pyramid for good health. However, foods at the bottom of the Pyramid represent foundational foods; we need to eat larger amounts of these foods. Foods at the top of the Pyramid should be eaten in much smaller amounts because of their fat and sugar content.
Materials:	Make a large Food Pyramid bulletin board (see p. 312 in the textbook or Fig.4-1). Food magazines, scissors, paper, tacks
Initiation:	Explain that no single food contains all of the nutrients needed for living. Nutrients are the building materials found in food that help us grow, learn, and play. People need to eat many different foods to stay healthy.
Activity:	Have students cut out food pictures from magazines or draw their favorite foods. Students decide which food group their picture represents and place the pictures on the appropriate level of the Food Pyramid bulletin board.
Closure:	Ask why it is important to eat food from all six parts of the Food Pyramid? Why do they think breads and cereals are in the foundation and the largest part of the Pyramid? Why is the top of the Pyramid the smallest?

NUTRITION
PRIMARY LEVEL

Objective:	**Describes food combinations that provide a balanced diet.**
Level:	Grades 1 and 2
Title:	*Fill Your Plate*
Integration:	Art
Vocabulary:	Pyramid
Content	
Generalization:	We need to eat a variety of foods from all of the major food categories shown in the Food Pyramid for good health. A balanced diet includes a variety of foods from the five most nutritious food groups. Foods at the top of the Pyramid represent the sixth food grouping. Foods in this group should be eaten in much smaller amounts than those in the other groups because of their fat and sugar content.
Materials:	Food magazines, scissors, glue, paper plates, paper, crayons. Food Pyramid bulletin board (See p. 312 in text or Fig. 4-1.)
Initiation:	Divide class into teams of three students. Hand out magazines, scissors, glue, paper, crayons, and paper plates to each team of students. Ask them to review the Food Pyramid.
Activity:	Explain that students are to plan a meal that contains the five most important components of the Food Pyramid using pictures from the magazines. If they cannot find a particular food, they can draw a picture of it. The food pictures are to be arranged and glued to the paper plates.
Closure:	Ask each team of students to show their "meal" to the rest of the class and explain why they think it is nutritionally balanced.

NUTRITION
PRIMARY LEVEL

Objective:	**Identifies snack foods that are nutritious.**
Level:	Kindergarten
Title:	*Let's Scream for Ice Cream!*
Integration:	Science
Vocabulary:	None
Content	
Generalization:	Snack foods can contribute important nutrients, such as protein, vitamins, and minerals, if properly selected. Many snacks, including chips, candy, cakes, and cookies, offer few other nutrients besides fat and sugar. Ice cream can be considered a nutritious snack when made from recipes that are low in fat, such as ice cream made with some of the cream replaced with milk or ice milk. Since it is made with milk, it contains calcium; vitamins D, A, riboflavin (a B-vitamin), and protein. Making ice cream also shows children that when salt is added to ice, it keeps the ice from melting at classroom temperature, so it remains cold enough to help make the ice cream.
Materials:	Electric or hand-crank ice cream maker, instructions, a recipe, and ingredients to make a batch of vanilla ice cream/ice milk for the class. Also needed are plastic spoons and small paper cups.
Initiation:	A few days in advance, tell the children that "Ice Cream Day" is coming. A field trip to a dairy farm may be conducted before the preparation of classroom ice cream.
Activity:	Make the ice cream or ice milk, following the directions. Serve.
Closure:	Ask children what makes ice cream or ice milk a good snack.

NUTRITION
PRIMARY LEVEL

Objective: **Identifies snack foods that are nutritious.**

Level: Kindergarten and grade 1

Title: *Fruit Snacks*

Integration: Reading readiness

Vocabulary: Nutritious, vitamin, kiwifruit, papaya, pomegranate, casaba melon, banana, pineapple, grapefruit

Content Generalization: Fruits are excellent choices for snacks. Most fruits are low in fat and good sources of vitamins A and C and the antioxidant nutrient, beta carotene.

Materials: Knife, paper towels, kiwifruit, papaya, pomegranate, casaba melon, grapefruit, banana, pineapple, small paper cups, plastic spoons, large bowl

Initiation: Write the names for the various fruits on the chalkboard. Place fruit where it is visible. Ask children to name each of the fruits, and point to the name of the fruit on the chalkboard

Activity: Peel and cut fruit into bite-size pieces. Make a fruit salad, and distribute samples in cups for each of the children.

Closure: Ask children if they know why fruit is a healthier snack than cookies or chips.

NUTRITION
INTERMEDIATE LEVEL

Objective: **Identifies factors that influence personal food choices.**

Level: Grades 5 and 6

Title: *Our Nation's Food Heritage*

Integration: Geography, social studies, language arts

Vocabulary: Heritage

Content Generalization: The United States is a "melting pot" of people from many countries who brought with them their various cultural heritages. Many of our favorite foods and spices were introduced into this country by the many cultures represented by immigrants. Hot Mexican dishes, spicy curries, many "deli" foods, Chinese stir-fry, and Italian pastas have become part of modern American food preferences. When studying various countries, teachers can include information about the foods of nations.

Materials: Maps, electric cook-top and other cooking utensils (if necessary)

Initiation: Have students identify people in the school or community who are from another country. Have students prepare invitations to ask them to come to the classroom and present information about their country and its foods. Ask the guest to wear native clothes and prepare a native food, if possible.

Activity: Have the guests spend about 45 minutes describing their country's traditions and foods. Allow time for students to ask guests questions.

Closure: Ask students to compose thank you notes to the guest speakers highlighting what they learned about the origin of some of their food preferences.

NUTRITION
INTERMEDIATE LEVEL

Objective:	**Classifies foods according to their major nutrients.**
Level:	Grades 5 and 6
Title:	*FoodGo*
Integration:	Language arts
Vocabulary:	None
Content Generalization:	Foods can be classified by their major nutrient contribution. Some foods are more nutritious than others. For example, liver, eggs, and milk are major contributors of protein, various vitamins, and minerals. Other foods are more limited in their nutritional contribution to the diet; for example, sugar and oil are nearly 100% carbohydrate and 100% fat, respectively.
Materials:	FoodGo game boards and game chips (See Fig.4-2 for instructions.) Food composition tables, water-soluble marking pens, fish bowl.
Initiation:	Divide class into teams. Provide food composition tables, a FoodGo game board, and envelope with nutrient chips for each group.
Activity:	Explain that the game is played like bingo. The teacher shuffles the nutrient role cards and then picks a card. After the teacher reads the nutrient role card to the class, students work together to decide if a food group is a major source of that nutrient. If it is, they find the appropriate nutrient chip in the envelope and place it on the appropriate space on the game board. Some of the nutrients have more that one function or are found in more than one food grouping. The first group to complete a row, column, or diagonal row calls "FoodGo!" The teacher and class review the winning team's choices to decide if they have made the correct food choices. If another team successfully challenges the winning team's choices, the winning team loses its winner status and must return the chip in question to the envelope. The game continues until a team correctly matches nutrients with food groups and functions.
Closure:	Ask "losing" team students to choose a nutrient and write a one-page essay identifying foods rich in that particular nutrient.

NUTRITION
INTERMEDIATE LEVEL

Objective: **Analyzes the nutritional value of food choices for meals and snacks.**

Level: Grades 5 and 6

Title: *Learning From Labels*

Integration: Math

Vocabulary: Calories

Content Generalization: The nutritional information on labels provides valuable information for consumers to use when comparing the nutritional value of products. Information about caloric value and percentages of daily values for key nutrients are given.

Materials: 50 different empty food packages that have nutritional labeling. Poster of food label (See p. 397 of textbook.)

Initiation: Place food label poster where it is visible. Ask students to choose a partner. Give each pair of students two of the empty food packages.

Activity: Using the poster, explain how one can use the label to judge the nutritional value of the product. Have students decide which of their products is the best source of iron, protein, and calcium. Ask them to identify which product is lower in Calories per serving. What is the serving size? Ask them to calculate the percentage of each product's total Calories that is contributed by fat. Which product contributes the greater percentage of fat?

Closure: Ask each student to bring in an empty food package from home. They should find a food product that has less than 30% of its total Calories from fat.

NUTRITION
INTERMEDIATE LEVEL

Objective: **Explains reasons for differences in nutritional requirements between individuals.**

Level: Grades 5 and 6

Title: *A Day in the Life of Joe and Wes*

Integration: Math

Vocabulary: Lifestyles, Calories

Content Generalization: Youngsters make choices concerning their activity patterns. Some choose to be active, others inactive. Inactive lifestyles are more likely to lead to the development of excess body fat, since there is less need for food energy to fuel activity. The excess food energy (Calories) is converted to body fat and stored for future use. Therefore one reason why individuals' needs for food energy varies is their different activity levels.

Materials: Handout (Fig. 4-3) A Day in the Life of Joe and Wes. Key to Handout (Fig. 4-4). 1 pound chunk of beed fat with any meat trimmed away

Initiation: Place the 1 pound chunk of fat where it is visible. Explain that it weighs 1 pound and that human fat is similar. Each pound of body fat represents an excess of 3500 Calories of food energy that is stored for future energy needs.

Activity: Give students the handout to determine the differences in Joe's and Wes's lifestyles.

Closure: What is one reason why people can differ in their caloric needs?

NUTRITION
MIDDLE SCHOOL LEVEL

Objective: **Evaluates diets appropriate for individual needs.**

Level: Grades 6 and 7

Title: *Menu-trition*

Integration: Analysis

Vocabulary: None

Content Generalization: We need to eat a variety of foods from all of the major food categories shown in the Food Pyramid for good health. A balanced diet includes a variety of foods from the five most nutritious food groups. Foods at the top of the Pyramid represent the sixth food grouping. Foods in this group should be eaten in much smaller amounts than those in the other groups because of their fat and sugar content.

Materials: Food Pyramid poster made from heavy cardboard (See p. 312 in textbook or Fig. 4-1.) Handout (Fig. 4-5) Menu Guides

Initiation: Place Food Pyramid poster where it is visible. Hand out menus.

Activity: Ask students to design a menu that includes foods they like to eat and meets the minimum number of servings as recommended by the Food Pyramid guide.

Closure: Ask students to explain why the Food Pyramid food guide is useful for menu planning.

NUTRITION
MIDDLE SCHOOL LEVEL

Objective:	**Explains the relationship between caloric intake, level of activity, and body weight.**
Level:	Grades 7 and 8
Title:	*Calories In, Calories Out*
Integration:	Math, analysis
Vocabulary:	Calories, energy balance
Content Generalization:	The concept of energy balance involves managing body fat levels through manipulating caloric intake and expenditure. Physical activity is a major way that Calories are used by the body. Body weight is maintained when caloric intake (food) equals caloric output (energy use by the body). Body fat represents stored energy. Each pound of fat represents about 3500 Calories. When a person gains a pound, they have consumed 3500 more Calories than needed to fuel body activities. If their energy needs are greater than their caloric (energy) intake, they will lose weight. Weight loss or gain takes place over time. On some days, people may have an excess of Calories (+); on other days, they may not have eaten enough (-). When the excess or deficit reaches a total of 3500 Calories, a gain or loss of 1 pound of body weight can be expected.
Materials:	Handout (Fig. 4-6) A Week's Worth of Differences, Key to A Week's Worth of Differences (Fig.4-7)
Initiation:	Ask if any students have tried to lose or gain weight. What did they do to accomplish weight gain or loss? Were they successful? Explain concept of energy balance.
Activity:	Give handouts to students. Ask them to compare each day's total Calorie intake to expenditure and determine if there was an excess (+) or a deficit (-) of Calories. After analyzing each day of the week, students should be able to determine if this person would be expected to gain or lose weight or stay at the same weight.
Closure:	Ask students to explain why the person would not be expected to gain or lose a pound of body fat. What role does physical activity play in altering body fat levels?

NUTRITION
MIDDLE SCHOOL LEVEL

Objective:	**Analyzes nutritional value of food in fad diets.**
Level:	Grades 6 through 8
Title:	Diet Plan Roulette
Integration:	Science, analysis
Vocabulary:	Fad

Content

Generalization: A fad is something that is fashionable for a time. Fad weight-loss diets promise quick and easy weight reduction. Gimmicks, such as eating an unusual type of food or using a device to "rub" fat away, are often included. People will lose weight on these diets because they restrict total caloric intake. However, people often become bored with the plans and return to their former eating behaviors. At worst, people may become ill on the most restrictive of the diets. One can test a weight reduction plan to determine if it is reasonable and safe. Does it include foods from all of the food groups? Does it include a plan to increase physical activity? Does it include foods that are familiar and available to the individual? Does it avoid making any promises or gimmicks? Does it lead to gradual, steady weight loss? Can one follow this plan for a lifetime? The answers should be yes to all of these questions.

Materials: Handout (Fig. 4-8) Marta's Latest Weight Loss Diet. Key to Marta's Latest Weight Loss Diet (Fig. 4-9) Pyramid Poster (Fig. 4-1)

Initiation: Ask, "How many of you have tried to lose or gain weight?" "How did you attempt to do this?" "Were you successful?" List the characteristics of a reasonable weight reduction diet on the chalkboard.

Activity: Give students a copy of the handout. Ask them to analyze the diet plan using the list and the recommendations of the Food Pyramid. They should decide if it is a reasonable weight loss plan or an example of a fad diet.

Closure: Ask students what characteristics can be used to determine if a diet is a fad.

NUTRITION
MIDDLE SCHOOL LEVEL

Objective:	**Predicts long-range outcomes of poor diet choices.**
Level:	Grades 7 and 8
Title:	*Mice Experiment*
Integration:	Science, observation, prediction
Vocabulary:	Control, experimental
Content	
Generalization:	Poor dietary choices lead to nutritional problems, including excess body fat, poor growth, and other signs of ill health.
Materials:	Six young mice from the same litter, two aquariums, three food dishes, water bottles, commercial mouse food, candy bars, cookies, cakes, sawdust chips, gram balance, record books
Initiation:	Explain that the purpose of this study is to observe any changes in the mice after they follow two different diets for a 3-week period. Ask students to design a study using six mice to compare the effects of a diet high in fat and sugar with a diet formulated especially to meet the dietary needs of mice. They should determine that one group of three mice (control) will be kept in an aquarium and fed mice food from a bowl. The second group of mice (experimental) will be kept in the other aquarium but will be fed cookies, candy, and other sweets. The experimental group should **also** be given a bowl of mice food. Both mice groups need to have adequate water.
Activity:	Have students identify each aquarium as "control" or "experimental." Students can be divided into two teams. One will measure and observe the control mice; the other will measure and observe the experimental mice. Each mouse needs to have its weight recorded at the start of the study. Each group provides the diet for their mice and is responsible for keeping the mice environment clean. Food needs to be replaced daily, **including** weekends. Students should observe and record any changes in mouse behavior, weight, and appearance. Weigh each mouse every other day. At the end of the three-week study, students in each team should analyze the data collected and come to some conclusion about the effects of each type of diet on a mouse. Ask one student from each team to write mice weights and any other significant observations about the mice in their group on the board. Have students compare findings.
Closure:	Ask, "What can you determine about a diet high in fat and sugar for the health of mice?" "What do you think happens to humans who eat this kind of diet?"

Obtain a veterinarian's and administrative approval before beginning this study. Certain animal studies may not be permissible in your district. Before the study, determine where mice will go when the study is completed.

DISEASE PREVENTION AND CONTROL
Student Objectives

Primary Level K-3 Student:

1.   Explains differences between illness and wellness.
2.   Differentiates between infectious and other diseases.
3.   Identifies ways to prevent the spread of disease.
4.   Explains the importance of health checkups and immunization to health maintenance.

Intermediate Level 4-5/6 Student:

1.   Identifies factors that may cause diseases and disorders.
2.   Differentiates between control of infectious and other diseases.
3.   Explains the contribution of science to the detection, prevention, and control of disease.

Middle School Level 6/7-8 Student:

1.   Analyzes the relationship of personal lifestyle choices to disease prevention.
2.   Identifies the symptoms of diseases common among young people.
3.   Explains the effects of disease on individuals, families, and communities.
4.   Describes appropriate courses of action when a disease is suspected.

DISEASE PREVENTION AND CONTROL
PRIMARY LEVEL

Objective:	**Explains the difference between illness and wellness.**
Level:	Kindergarten
Title:	*When I Am Sick*
Integration:	Reading readiness, art, comparison
Vocabulary:	Ill, well
Content Generalization:	Individual health varies from day to day. When one is ill, he or she feels different and uncomfortable. The person may show signs of illness, such as having a rash or a fever.
Materials:	Handout (Fig. 5-1) When I Am Sick, crayons
Initiation:	Write the words "ill" and "well" on the chalkboard. Ask children do they feel well now or ill (sick)? How do they know when they are well or sick?
Activity:	Give children the handout, and ask them to draw two pictures of themselves. One picture is what they look like when they feel well and on the other side, when they feel ill.
Closure:	Ask children to show their pictures. Do they see any that look almost the same? What is the difference between being well and being ill?

DISEASE PREVENTION AND CONTROL
PRIMARY LEVEL

Objective:	**Differentiates between infectious and other diseases.**
Level:	Grade 3
Title:	*I Can Catch A Cold*
Integration:	Science, language arts, comparison
Vocabulary:	Germs, infectious diseases, noninfectious diseases, lifestyle
Content Generalization:	Some diseases are caused by infectious agents, such as bacteria and viruses (germs). People vary in their ability to avoid becoming ill when they come into contact with infectious agents. Their immune systems may be able to prevent the infectious agent from causing illness. Others become sick but may get better over time. In other cases, there are no treatments for the illness and people may not live. Noninfectious diseases are illnesses not caused by infectious agents but that generally result from the way the person chooses to live, their lifestyle. The diseases of lifestyle include lung cancer resulting from cigarette smoking or high blood pressure resulting from being overweight. Heart disease and strokes have a very strong link to lifestyle choices, such as smoking, eating a high-fat diet, and not exercising.
Initiation:	Ask the librarian to locate some books about diseases for the class to use, and place them in a special area. Set a date to bring the class to the library for research. Write the terms "infectious diseases," "noninfectious diseases," and "lifestyle" on the chalkboard. Ask students if they can think of the differences between the two major types of diseases. What role does lifestyle play in becoming sick? Ask class if they know someone who is sick. Do they have an infectious disease or a noninfectious one? How can they tell?
Activity:	Assign students to work in teams to research one of the following diseases: lung cancer, hepatitis, cirrhosis, high blood pressure, tuberculosis, influenza, heart disease, strokes, diabetes, AIDS, lyme disease, and colds. They are to go to the library, find information about the disease, and write a two-page paper. These papers will be read to the class by one of the students in the team. Take the class to the library for the first research session. Give students about 5 days to prepare disease reports.
Closure:	After the disease reports have been given, ask students if they can classify each of the diseases as infectious (I) or noninfectious (N). Lung cancer (N), hepatitis (usually I), cirrhosis (usually N), high blood pressure (N), tuberculosis (I), influenza (I), heart disease (usually N), strokes (N), diabetes (N), AIDS (I), lyme disease (I), and colds (I)

DISEASE PREVENTION AND CONTROL
PRIMARY LEVEL

Objective:	**Identifies ways to prevent the spread of disease.**
Level:	Grade 3
Title:	*Stopping the Spread*
Integration:	Science
Vocabulary:	Infectious disease, immunization, vaccine
Content Generalization:	Many infectious diseases can be prevented or controlled. Vaccines have been developed to prevent infectious diseases, such as whooping cough, diphtheria, polio and tetanus. Adequate community sanitation as well as personal hygiene practices are also important ways to control the spread of infectious disease. Individuals need to remember to wash their hands after going to the bathroom, handling soiled materials, and playing with pets. Wash hands before preparing food and eating and after coughing or blowing one's nose. Don't share food utensils or eat from other's plates. Avoid contact with another person's body fluids, such as blood.
Initiation:	Write the words "immunization" and "vaccine" on the chalkboard. Ask children if they have seen their immunization records. Do they know what immunization means? Why are people immunized?
Activity:	Brainstorm other ways that diseases can be prevented, giving emphasis to personal hygienic practices. Write their suggestions on the board.
Closure:	Ask children which disease prevention practices will they focus on while at home and school?

DISEASE PREVENTION AND CONTROL
PRIMARY LEVEL

Objective:	**Explains the importance of health checkups and immunizations to health maintenance.**
Level:	Grade 1
Title:	*Bears Need Doctors, Too*
Integration:	Science
Vocabulary:	Doctor
Content Generalization:	Regular health check-ups are important because medical practitioners can detect and treat illnesses early, provide immunizations and record growth and development. When established early in life, these preventive behaviors are more likely to continue for a lifetime. Children often associate going to the doctor with when they are sick or need an immunization. It's important for them to recognize that even when you feel fine, future problems can be detected and growth can be checked.
Materials:	Toy car, book: *The Berenstain Bears Go to the Doctor*, Stan and Janice Berenstain, Random House, New York, 1981 (ISBN 0-394-94835-1)
Initiation:	Ask children to sit in preparation for "storytelling" time. Show the toy car and ask children, "What do your parents do to keep their car running just right?" "Do they take it anywhere for checkups (oil changes, tune-ups, etc.)?" People are like cars; they need checkups too. Ask, "Where do people go for check-ups?" "What do doctors do when they give a checkup?"
Activity:	Read the story to the children.
Closure:	Ask children, "Why do we need regular medical checkups?

DISEASE PREVENTION AND CONTROL
INTERMEDIATE LEVEL

Objective:	**Identifies factors that may cause diseases and disorders.**
Level:	Grades 4 and 5
Title:	*My Family's Medical History*
Integration:	Science
Vocabulary:	Heredity, infectious and noninfectious diseases, bacteria, viruses
Content Generalization:	Some diseases are caused by infectious agents, such as bacteria, viruses, and parasites. People vary in their ability to avoid becoming ill when they come into contact with infectious agents (germs). Their immune systems may be able to prevent the infectious agent from causing illness. Others become sick but may get better over time. In other cases, there are no treatments for the illness, and people may not live. Noninfectious diseases are illnesses not caused by infectious agents. People may be born with a condition, such as cystic fibrosis. This is an example of an inherited disorder that one cannot control. However, the majority of noninfectious diseases generally result from the way the person chooses to live, their lifestyle. The lifestyle diseases include most cancers such as lung cancer that results from cigarette smoking or high blood pressure that results from being overweight. Heart disease and strokes have a very strong link to lifestyle choices, such as smoking, eating a high-fat diet, and not exercising.
Materials:	None
Initiation:	Write the words "infectious disease" and "noninfectious disease" on the chalkboard. Ask children to identify the difference between these diseases.
Activity:	Ask students to discuss their family history with parents. What kinds of diseases did their grandparents suffer from? Were they infectious or non-infectious? What may have caused their diseases? Students are to write a paragraph about their family's medical history and what may have caused the illnesses experienced by their family members.
Closure:	Ask students to list the various causes of diseases.

DISEASE PREVENTION AND CONTROL
INTERMEDIATE LEVEL

Objective:	**Differentiates between control of infectious and other diseases.**
Level:	Grades 7 and 8
Title:	*Century of Change*
Integration:	Language arts, science
Vocabulary:	Immunizations, vaccine, antibiotics
Content Generalization:	Since 1900, medical advancements have be able to prevent or control many infectious diseases. Vaccines have been developed to prevent whooping cough, diphtheria, polio, and tetanus. Antibiotics have been discovered to treat infectious diseases that used to be deadly. Better nutrition, improved community sanitation facilities, and education about personal hygiene have helped to control the spread of infectious diseases. Today, the majority of deaths are caused by noninfectious diseases. These diseases generally result from the way a person chooses to live, their lifestyle. Lifestyle diseases include lung cancer that results from cigarette smoking or high blood pressure that results from being overweight. Heart disease and strokes have a very strong link to lifestyle choices, such as smoking, eating a high-fat diet, and not exercising. Controlling these diseases involves education and behavioral change.
Materials:	None
Initiation:	Ask students to list ways infectious and noninfectious diseases are controlled.
Activity:	Ask students to write an essay on the changes in the causes of death from 1900 to the present. What factors account for this change in the nature of the cause of death?
Closure:	Ask, "What can we do to control today's more serious diseases?"

DISEASE PREVENTION AND CONTROL
INTERMEDIATE LEVEL

Objective: **Identifies ways to prevent the spread of disease.**

Level: Grade 6

Title: *The Prevention Challenge*

Integration: Science

Vocabulary: None

Content Generalization: The spread of many infectious diseases can be prevented or controlled. Vaccines have been developed to prevent influenza, whooping cough, diphtheria, polio, and tetanus. Adequate community sanitation as well as personal hygiene practices are also important ways to control the spread of infectious disease. Individuals need to remember to wash their hands after going to the bathroom, handling soiled materials, and playing with pets. Wash hands before preparing food and eating and after coughing or blowing one's nose. Don't share food utensils or eat from other's plates. Avoid contact with another person's body fluids, such as blood.

Materials: Paper and pencil

Initiation: Divide class into two teams. Have them move their seats to opposite ends of the classroom.

Activity: Tell each team to remain quiet. At the moment the teacher tells them to begin, students are to list as many ways as they can that the spread of diseases can be prevented. At the end of 5 minutes, teams turn in their lists to the teacher. The team with the most ideas obtains 5 bonus points.

Closure: The teacher shares the winning team's list with the class and compares it to the others'.

DISEASE PREVENTION AND CONTROL
INTERMEDIATE LEVEL

Objective: **Explains the contribution of science to the detection, prevention, and control of disease.**

Level: Grades 7 and 8

Title: *Medical Miracle Workers*

Integration: Science, language arts, analysis

Vocabulary: Epidemiologists, epidemiology

Content Generalization: Many scientists have contributed to the detection of disease-causing agents, prevention of disease, and its control. Some scientists discovered the agents of disease, others determined effective treatments, and still others found ways to prevent its spread. Epidemiology is the study of the factors that contribute to and spread disease. Current research involves understanding how viruses can be controlled and developing effective antiviral agents.

Materials: None

Initiation: Make an appointment to take the class to the library. Have a librarian review features of the library, including how to locate information.

Activity: Students are to choose one scientist who made a contribution to disease prevention and control, read about their efforts, and write a three page paper about their contribution to society. Possible choices include Jenner, Virchow, Lister, the Curies, Fleming, Florey, Reed, Pasteur, Koch, Sabin, and Salk.

Closure: Ask students what makes their scientist's contribution to society so important?

DISEASE PREVENTION AND CONTROL
INTERMEDIATE LEVEL

Objective:	**Demonstrates how HIV infection affects the functioning of the immune system.**
Level:	Grades 5 and 6
Title:	*Immune Buster*
Integration:	Science
Vocabulary:	Immune system, opportunistic diseases, HIV, AIDS
Content Generalization:	HIV infection can disable the immune system, rendering it unable to prevent infectious diseases from causing illness. When this occurs, the person develops opportunistic infections, such as TB and certain cancers that a normal immune system would prevent. This results in the deadly disease, AIDS.
Materials:	Notecards, marking pens, yarn, several blindfolds
Initiation:	Explain how HIV causes AIDS by disabling the immune system. Have children take the notecards and write the following names: HIV, immune cell, TB bacteria cell, flu virus, and chickenpox virus. Punch holes in the namecards, and string yarn through to make necklaces. Ask children to pick a "role," for example, someone to play HIV and so on. Mark off part of the classroom as "inside" the body and another part as outside the body. Have children who are playing infectious agents stand on the "outside" of the body and the immune system cells stand inside the body.
Activity:	Children demonstrate how a healthy body's immune system cells handle infectious agents when they try to gain entry into the body part of the classroom. (The immune cells remove the infectious agents' nametags to show that the agents are being destroyed.) To demonstrate how HIV works to disable the immune cells, have the HIV students enter the body part of the classroom and place blindfolds over the eyes of the immune system cell actors. Now that the immune cells cannot see what is happening, the other infectious agents can enter without being destroyed. The person develops a variety of serious illnesses that a healthy immune system would prevent. These illnesses are called opportunistic because they are taking advantage of the disabled immune system.
Closure:	Ask students if they can explain why people with HIV do not die directly from the virus.

66

DISEASE PREVENTION AND CONTROL
MIDDLE SCHOOL LEVEL

Objective: **Analyzes the relationship of personal lifestyle choices to disease prevention.**

Level: Grades 7 and 8

Title: *Lifestyle Game*

Integration: Science

Vocabulary: Intravenous, cirrhosis

Content Generalization: Today, the majority of deaths are caused by noninfectious diseases. These diseases generally result from the way a person chooses to live, their lifestyle. Cigarette smoking is a behavior that has been linked to many diseases including lung cancer, hypertension, heart disease, and strokes. Excess body fat, which results from poor dietary choices and lack of physical activity, contributes to heart disease, hypertension, and diabetes. Sexually transmitted diseases result from unprotected sexual activity. AIDS can result from sharing needles when abusing intravenous drugs. Serious liver diseases, such as cirrhosis often result from alcohol abuse. Controlling these diseases involves education and behavioral change.

Materials: Three sets of notecards with each of the following terms written on them: smoking, sexual intercourse, alcohol abuse, "couch potato," high fat diet, excess body fat, lung cancer, cirrhosis, AIDS, sexually transmitted disease, heart disease, stroke, and diabetes. Place each set of notecards in an envelope.

Initiation: Before this activity, make certain that every student has returned the parental permission form (a sample letter is shown on p. 305). For those students who did not obtain parental OK, excuse them from the class. Give them a project concerning disease prevention and control that requires library work. Ask students to divide up into three teams. Give each team an envelope. Students are to work in teams to match diseases with lifestyle behaviors. Tell them it is possible to have more than one disease matching a particular lifestyle. It is also possible to more than one lifestyle contributing to a disease.

Closure: After about 15 minutes, ask each group to report on their matches. All teams should agree that the matches are correct.

DISEASE PREVENTION AND CONTROL
MIDDLE SCHOOL LEVEL

Objective:	**Analyzes the relationship of personal lifestyle choices to disease prevention.**
Level:	Grade 8
Title:	*Be My Friend*
Integration:	Social studies, science
Vocabulary:	Infectious disease, sexually transmitted diseases (STD), gonorrhea, syphilis, chlamydia, genital herpes, AIDS
Content Generalization:	Sexually transmitted diseases usually result from unprotected sexual activity. The most reliable way to prevent infection with an STD is to avoid sexual intercourse. For those who choose not to abstain from sexual intercourse, avoiding casual sexual encounters can reduce one's risk of contracting an STD. Controlling these diseases involves education and behavioral change.
Materials:	**Obtain administrative approval** to discuss STD. 40 painted tongue-depressors (8 blue, 8 red, 8 silver, 8 green, and 8 gold)
Initiation:	Tell students that it's time to play the Be My Friend game. Give 5 boys and girls a set of 8 colored tongue-depressors of the same color.
Activity:	Tell the students with the tongue-depressors begin the game by walking around the room and choosing a person to get to know. They should explore the possibility of becoming friends. If the students with tongue-depressors decide that they want to become another student's friend, they are to give them a tongue-depressor. If the other person does not want to be their friend, they do not accept the tongue-depressor. This friendship activity continues for 15-20 minutes. As soon as any individual has two of the same colored tongue-depressors, they can try to meet someone and exchange tongue-depressors. The rules are that a student cannot exchange tongue-depressors until they have two of the same color and they always keep one of each color they have received. At the end of the time allotted, ask, "How many students do not have any tongue-depressors?" "How many have more than one color?"

On the chalkboard, write: Sexually Transmitted Diseases (STD)

Blue = gonorrhea
Red = syphilis
Green = chlamydia
Silver = genital herpes
Gold = AIDS

Ask students if they can explain what the game represented. (Every time they decided to give a tongue-depressor and the other person accepted it,

68

they were transmitting an STD. The game demonstrates how casual sexual encounters spread STD)

Closure: Ask, "What is the best way to avoid an STD?"

DISEASE PREVENTION AND CONTROL
MIDDLE SCHOOL LEVEL

Objective:	**Identifies symptoms of diseases common among young people.**
Title:	*STD ID*
Level:	Grades 7 and 8
Integration:	Science
Vocabulary:	STD, gonorrhea, syphilis, chlamydia, HIV/AIDS, genital herpes, genital warts, cervical cancer
Content Generalization:	Rates of sexually transmitted diseases among young people are increasing as they become more sexually active. Symptoms such as sores, growths, blisters, pain, or discharge are noticeable. Other symptoms may be unnoticed and cause damage to the brain and reproductive organs. Recognizing the long-term social and physical consequences of these diseases is important. The most reliable form of prevention is sexual abstinence.
Materials:	Parental approval letters, drawing or slides of physical signs of STD (available from Planned Parenthood education centers), slide projector
Initiation:	Inform your administrator about the content of this activity and that it meets the above objective. **Obtain administrative approval.** Invite parents to attend the class. Before this activity, make certain that every student has returned the parental permission form (a sample letter is shown on p. 305). For those students who did not obtain parental OK, excuse them from the class. Give them a project concerning disease prevention and control that requires library work. Invite school nurse into the classroom to answer students' questions about STD.
Activity:	Show drawings or slides of physical signs of STD. Have the nurse answer student questions about physical and social effects, such as impaired fertility, increased risk of cervical cancer, birth defects, and infant deaths.
Closure:	Ask students if they can identify the only 100% effective way to prevent an STD.

DISEASE PREVENTION AND CONTROL
MIDDLE SCHOOL LEVEL

Objective:	**Explains the effects of disease on individuals, families, and communities.**
Level:	Grades 7 and 8
Title:	*The AIDS Tragedy*
Integration:	Social studies
Vocabulary:	None
Content Generalization:	The AIDS epidemic is touching virtually every community. Its cost to society in medical and social terms is enormous, but it is devastating to families. Adolescents often take an "it won't happen to me" approach to risky behaviors. Seeing an individual with this disease and talking to them and their loved ones will be a memorable experience.
Materials:	Parental approval letters
Initiation:	Inform your administrator about the nature and content of this activity and that it meets the above objective. Obtain administrative approval. Invite a person with AIDS to come to the class along with one of his or her close family members. Explain to them the objective of the lesson. Before this activity, make certain that every student has returned the parental permission form (a sample letter is shown on p. 305). For those students who did not obtain parental OK, excuse them from the class. Give them a project concerning disease prevention and control that requires library work. Invite parents to this class. Invite school nurse into the classroom to answer students' questions about HIV/AIDS. Students are to prepare a set of questions to ask the guests.
Activity:	Arrange seating informally. Have the person with AIDS describe his or her condition and the effects this disease has had on them and their family. Permit students to ask questions at any time during their presentation.
Closure:	Ask students to write thank-you notes to send to the guests. The notes should mention what they have learned about AIDS, particularly how it affects everyone.

DISEASE PREVENTION AND CONTROL
MIDDLE SCHOOL LEVEL

Objective:	**Describes appropriate courses of action when a disease is suspected.**
Level:	Grades 7 and 8
Title:	*When Am I Too Sick?*
Integration:	Science, language arts
Vocabulary:	Signs, symptoms
Content Generalization:	In many cases, self-care of illness is the appropriate course of action; at other times, it is crucial to obtain prompt emergency care. Being able to recognize when one is sick enough to seek medical care is an important skill. Certain signs (physically apparent conditions) and symptoms (reported sensations) are useful when determining how ill an individual is.
Materials:	None
Initiation:	Invite school nurse into classroom as guest speaker. Write the words "signs" and "symptoms" on the board. Ask students if they know the difference.
Activity:	Have the school nurse present information concerning the evaluation of various physical signs and symptoms of illness, such as fever, sore throat, diarrhea, vomiting, rashes, and headaches. Ask the nurse to address when signs and symptoms signify a potentially serious condition. For example, at what point do you contact a physician for vomiting?
Closure:	Have students investigate various effective self-care treatments for each of the listed illness signs and symptoms. They should determine when self-care for the condition should be discontinued and expert medical advice sought.

INJURY PREVENTION AND SAFETY
Student Objectives

Primary Level K-3 Student:

1. Explains the relationship between observing safety rules and preventing injuries.
2. Identifies potential hazards at home, school, and community.
3. Explains how to obtain help in an emergency.

Intermediate Level 4-5/6 Student:

1. Evaluates actions of bicycle riders for safety.
2. Demonstrates basic first aid procedures for stopped breathing.
3. Identifies individual responsibilities for reducing hazards and preventing injuries.

Middle School Level 6/7-8 Student:

1. Develops a home safety program.
2. Demonstrates standard first aid procedures appropriate in life-threatening situations.
3. Explains how properly used protective equipment increases enjoyment and diminishes the possibility of injury when engaging in potentially risky activities.

INJURY PREVENTION AND SAFETY
PRIMARY LEVEL

Objective: **Explains the relationship between observing safety rules and preventing injuries.**

Level: Kindergarten and grade 1

Title: *Dinosaurs, Beware*

Integration: Reading readiness

Vocabulary: Safety

Content Generalization: Rules of safety involve following certain practices that reduce the risk of injury or death. By learning these rules and having opportunities to practice them, youngsters can increase their sense of control over their personal safety.

Materials: Book: *Dinosaurs, Beware!* by Marc Brown and Stephen Krensky, Little, Brown & Company, Boston, 1982. (ISBN: 0-316-11228-3)

Initiation: Have children prepare move their seats into position for "storytelling time."

Activity: Read book to children, and show pictures.

Closure: Ask children, "What was your favorite dinosaur safety behavior?"

INJURY PREVENTION AND SAFETY
PRIMARY LEVEL

Objective:	**Explains the relationship between observing safety rules and preventing injuries.**
Level:	Kindergarten and grade 1
Title:	*Stop, Drop, and Roll*
Integration:	Language arts, science
Vocabulary:	Stop, drop, roll, fire
Content Generalization:	Rules of safety involve following certain practices that reduce the risk of injury or death. By learning these rules and having opportunities to practice them, youngsters can increase their sense of control over their personal safety.
Materials:	None
Initiation:	Take a field trip to the firehouse. Write "stop," "drop," and "roll" on the chalkboard. Have children read the words. Arrange desks so that there is a large open area in the classroom. Ask children if they have ever watched an adult trying to light a charcoal grill or a fireplace. Did the adult have to "fan" the fire to make it burn more?
Activity:	Demonstrate what you should do if your clothes catch on fire (stop moving, drop to the ground, and roll around). Explain to children that if they try to run, they will become more hurt by the fire. Air "fans" a fire, making it burn hotter.
Closure:	Have children practice, one at a time, what they have memorized by saying "stop, drop, and roll!"

INJURY PREVENTION AND SAFETY
PRIMARY LEVEL

Objective:	**Identifies potential hazards at home, school and community.**
Level:	Kindergarten through grade 3
Title:	*Safe Smarts*
Integration:	Social studies, analysis
Vocabulary:	Stranger
Content Generalization:	Children are vulnerable. Teaching them basic safety rules to follow when they are not with adults they know and trust is crucial. They must understand that any teenager or adult who they do not know is a stranger and represents a danger to their safety.
Materials:	None
Initiation:	Write the word "stranger," on the chalkboard. Ask students to describe a stranger. Are they always creepy, evil-looking characters? Can strangers be teenagers?
Activity:	Invite a local policeman into the classroom to explain personal safety rules to children. For example, how do they respond to situations in which a friendly stranger asks for help or invites them into their car? What if they tell the child their parents said it was OK to go with them? What if the stranger grabs them and tries to force them into a car?
Closure:	Ask children what they should do if they are alone and someone offers to give them a ride home. What will they do if someone they don't know asks for help to find their lost puppy. What if someone says their mother is in the hospital and she told them to take you there?

INJURY PREVENTION AND SAFETY
PRIMARY LEVEL

Objective:	**Explains how to obtain help in an emergency.**
Level:	Kindergarten and grade 1
Title:	*Dialing for Help*
Integration:	Social studies
Vocabulary:	Address
Content Generalization:	Children should be able to recognize when and how to obtain help. Every child should learn their name, address and how to use an emergency access system, such as 911 or whatever is available in their community.
Materials:	Telephones (touch-tone and dial), home address list of students
Initiation:	Ask children to work in teams of three. Distribute telephones to each team. Write the word "address" on the chalkboard. Ask children if they know what the word means and if they know their own address. Ask each child to repeat their full name and address. If a child does not know their address, write it down for them, read it to them, and have them read it back to you. Tell them to practice giving their address to their teammates. Tell students that in an emergency, they can call for help. Give them the emergency access number. Ask students to describe situations that are emergencies.
Activity:	Have students practice using the telephone to dial for help.
Closure:	Ask students, "Now, what will you do if your mother falls down the steps and won't wake up?"

INJURY PREVENTION AND SAFETY
INTERMEDIATE

Objective:	**Evaluates actions of bicycle riders for safety.**
Level:	Grade 4
Title:	*Liking Biking*
Integration:	Social studies, observation
Vocabulary:	None
Content Generalization:	Every year, many youngsters are seriously injured or killed in accidents involving cars and bikes. Following basic bike safety rules and wearing helmets for head protection would help prevent many deaths and injuries. Youngsters also need to make certain that their bikes are in safe working condition.
Materials:	Child's bike, helmet
Initiation:	Invite a police officer into the classroom to present information concerning safe biking rules.
Activity:	Ask children to observe bicyclists in their community, including adults, for a week. Have them write a paragraph about the kinds of unsafe biking behaviors practiced by the bicyclists.
Closure:	Ask students, "What makes you a safe bike rider?"

INJURY PREVENTION AND SAFETY
INTERMEDIATE LEVEL

Objective:	**Demonstrates basic first aid procedures for stopped breathing.**
Level:	Grades 4 and 5
Title:	*Mr. Heimlich's Maneuver*
Integration:	Science
Vocabulary:	None
Content Generalization:	The Heimlich maneuver is an effective form of first aid for choking victims. By pushing forcibly on the diaphragm, air that is trapped in the lungs rushes out of the lungs with such force that it expels whatever is causing the choking.
Materials:	Lung chamber made from a plastic 2-liter bottle, latex glove, plastic stopper, glass "Y" tube or straws, 2 balloons, duct tape, and a piece of chewing gum (see Fig. 6-1), pillows
Initiation:	Show how the lungs work by pulling down on the latex diaphragm. Lightly place a piece of chewing gum over the "windpipe" to simulate choking. Try pulling down on the latex diaphragm; the balloons don't inflate since air can't enter the "lungs." Vigorously hit the latex diaphragm with your fist to dislodge the blockage. This demonstrates how the Heimlich maneuver saves people from choking. Invite the school nurse into the classroom to demonstrate ways to perform the Heimlich maneuver on people.
Activity:	Have children practice the Heimlich maneuver on the pillows.
Closure:	Role play situations with children in which they are eating and someone shows signs that they are choking. Have them act out what to do.

INJURY PREVENTION AND SAFETY
INTERMEDIATE

Objective: **Identifies individual responsibilities for reducing hazards and preventing injuries.**

Level: Grades 6 through 8

Title: *Safe at Play*

Integration: Social studies

Vocabulary: Paraplegic, quadriplegic

Content Generalization: Youngsters often take risks because they do not consider negative consequences of their behaviors. They often believe that nothing *bad* can happen to them. Playing is an enjoyable at any age, but youngsters need to be aware of what can happen if they don't use common sense and precautions. Some people become paraplegic or quadriplegic by breaking their necks in diving accidents; others are injured in biking or driving accidents.

Materials: Book: *Play it Safe: the kids' guide to personal safety and crime prevention,* Kathy S. Kyte, Alfred A. Knopf, Inc., New York, 1983 (ISBN 0-394-85964-2)

Initiation: Invite a person (paraplegic or quadriplegic) who has been severely injured while at play into the classroom. Explain to this individual that your intent is to make youngsters more aware of how actions can lead to unfortunate but preventable injuries. Be certain that the disabled individual is interested in helping youngsters appreciate the need for safety precautions.

Activity: Have the guest describe what they did that led to their condition. Allow students to ask questions concerning their recovery. (Explain that the guest is not expected to answer any questions that they think are embarrassing.)

Closure: Have students write a thank-you letter to the guest describing what they learned about taking precautions when at play. Assign students readings from the *Play it Safe* book. Have them select a type of safety concern, such as a home safety issue and write a one-page summary about how to protect oneself. Students will report to the rest of the class concerning their particular safety issue.

INJURY PREVENTION AND SAFETY
MIDDLE SCHOOL LEVEL

Objective:	**Develops a home safety program.**
Level:	Grades 6 and 7
Title:	*Getting Ready for the Big One*
Integration:	Science
Vocabulary:	Richter scale, seismic
Content Generalization:	Much of the United States has a potential for earthquake destruction. Preparation for threats to personal safety during and the lack of utilities after a major quake are important for people in these earthquake-prone areas.
Materials:	Seismic chart, map of North American earthquake risk zones, Red Cross earthquake disaster preparedness pamphlets.
Initiation:	As part of a physical science unit on the earth and its plate movements, discuss how the Richter scale indicates severity of an earthquake. Send a letter home explaining the activity to parents and requesting their cooperation.
Activity:	Have students research and develop an earthquake preparedness plan of action for their homes. The plan should include storing supplies, safety actions to take when an earthquake begins, and a plan to communicate with family members should they become separated. Parents need to review the plans with the student and indicate that they approve. Parents facilitate the preparedness and practice safety components of the plan.
Closure:	Have each student explain their plan to the rest of the class.

INJURY PREVENTION AND SAFETY
MIDDLE SCHOOL LEVEL

Objective:	**Demonstrates standard first aid procedures appropriate for life-threatening situations.**
Level:	Grades 6 through 8
Title:	*First Aid*
Integration:	Science
Vocabulary:	Resuscitation, Heimlich maneuver, hemorrhage
Content Generalization:	Being prepared to react appropriately in life-threatening situations is crucial. Basic first aid skills are necessary, as well as opportunities to practice these skills.
Materials:	Resuscitation doll, bleach water, paper towels, bandages (Ask guests to prepare a list of items needed for demonstrations.)
Initiation:	Send letter to parents to obtain permission for the class (see p.389 in text book). Ask students if they have ever been involved in an emergency situation. What happened? How did they react?
Activity:	Invite the school nurse or a Red Cross representative into the classroom to demonstrate proper first aid techniques, such as artificial respiration, the Heimlich maneuver, and control of severe bleeding.
Closure:	Give role-play situations to students that require first aid. For example, what would you do if you saw someone hit by a car?

INJURY PREVENTION AND SAFETY
MIDDLE SCHOOL LEVEL

Objective: **Explains how properly used protective equipment increases enjoyment and diminishes the possibility of injury when engaging in potentially risky activities.**

Level: Grades 6 through 8

Title: *Pumpkin-Head*

Integration: Science, prediction

Vocabulary: None

Content Generalization: Safety helmets are an extremely valuable piece of equipment. They are designed to take the force of a blow and distribute it through the helmet's construction materials and not to the skull and brain of the user.

Materials: 2 small pumpkins, hammer, youth's safety helmet, newspaper. Place pumpkins on newspaper where visible to students.

Initiation: Ask students to predict what will happen to the pumpkin "head" when it is hammered and unprotected by a helmet.

Activity: Demonstrate the value of a safety helmet by hitting an unprotected pumpkin with the hammer. Then hit the helmeted pumpkin with repeated blows. Remove the helmet to determine the extent of any damages. Have students examine the design of the helmet.

Closure: Students are to investigate proper safety equipment needs for one of their favorite activities, such as in-line skating, hockey, or football.

CONSUMER HEALTH
Student Objectives

Primary Level K-3 Student:

1. Differentiates between health products and services.
2. Names people who help promote health.
3. Explains the influence of advertising in promoting sale of health products.

Intermediate Level 4-5/6 Student:

1. Interprets information provided on health product labels.
2. Lists sources of reliable health information and services.
3. Describes advertising appeal of foods and medications used by children.
4. Differentiates between health quackery and licensed health care.

Middle School Level 6/7-8 Student:

1. Analyzes methods used to promote health products and services.
2. Compares scientific and faddish bases for choices among health products.
3. Describes the function of consumer-protection agencies.
4. Identifies criteria for the selection of a qualified health advisor.

CONSUMER HEALTH
PRIMARY LEVEL

Objective:	**Differentiates between health products and health services.**
Level:	Grade 2
Title:	*Do I Need This?*
Integration:	Language arts, art, analysis
Vocabulary:	Product, services
Content Generalization:	People are consumers of various health-care products and services. A health-care product is an item that is promoted to enhance health. A health-care service is an action performed by a specially trained individual that also contributes to health. The purchase of health-care services often involves buying related products as well. Not all health-care services or products are necessary. The purpose of advertising is to convince consumers the product or service is necessary, safe, and effective.
Materials:	Sample health product advertisement, magazines, scissors, paper, crayons.
Initiation:	Prepare blank bulletin board entitled, "Do I Need This?" Write "health-care product" and "health-care service" on the chalkboard. Ask students to define these terms and give examples. Show advertisement. Ask students to explain why products and services are advertised. Divide class into teams of students.
Activity:	Have each student team look for examples of health-care products or services in magazines. If they can not find a picture of a product or service, they are to draw and color some examples. Students make the bulletin board collage of their artwork and magazine clippings.
Closure:	Ask students to give an example of a health-care product and a health-care service.

CONSUMER HEALTH
PRIMARY LEVEL

Objective:	**Differentiates between health products and health services.**
Level:	Grade 3
Title:	*I Am a Consumer*
Integration:	Language arts, analysis
Vocabulary:	Consumer, product, services
Content	
Generalization:	People are consumers of various health-care products and services. A health-care product is an item that the consumer believes enhances health. A health-care service is an action performed by a specially trained individual that also contributes to health. The purchase of health-care services often involves buying related products as well. Not all health-care services or products are necessary.The purpose of advertising is to convince consumers the product or service is necessary, safe, and effective.
Materials:	Handout (Fig. 7-1) Health-Care Products at My House
Initiation:	Write "health-care products" and "health-care services" on the chalkboard. Ask students to explain the difference. Ask students to choose an example of a health-care product that is used at their home. Send a letter to parents explaining the need for examples of health-care products.
Activity:	Each child uses the handout to prepare a brief presentation about their health-care product. Why is it needed? How much does it cost? Why is this particular product bought rather than a similar one from another company?
Closure:	Ask students what influences people to purchase a particular health-care product or service.

CONSUMER HEALTH
PRIMARY LEVEL

Objective: **Names people who promote and protect health.**

Level: Grade 3

Title: *What's My Line?*

Integration: Social studies, analysis

Vocabulary: Occupations

Content Generalization: Many kinds of people work to prevent, control, and treat illnesses. Some of the more obvious health-care workers youngsters can identify are doctors and nurses. However others, such as pharmacists and food service establishment inspectors, play important health protection roles. Children need to recognize the variety of health-care occupations that exist.

Materials: Health worker ID cards (Fig. 7-2)

Initiation: Write "What's My Line?" on the chalkboard. Place two desks in the front of the classroom. One desk is for the student who plays the role of the game show host. The other desk is for the "health-care worker" guest.

Activity: Without informing the rest of the class, the host student picks another student to play the role of a health-care worker and shows the "worker" an ID card. The rest of the class asks questions about the worker's occupation to try to determine what it is. For example, students could ask, "Do you perform surgery?" The host guides the questioning. Once the occupation has been identified, the host writes the occupation on the chalkboard.

Closure: Ask students to list the kinds of workers who promote and protect health.

CONSUMER HEALTH
PRIMARY LEVEL

Objective: Explains the influence of advertising in promoting sales of health products.

Level: Grade 3

Title: *Buy This, Buy That*

Integration: Language arts, analysis

Vocabulary: Claims, testimonials

Content Generalization: People are consumers of various health-care products and services. A health-care product is an item that the consumer believes enhances health. A health-care service is an action performed by a specially trained individual that also contributes to health. The purchase of health-care services often involves buying related products as well. Not all health-care services or products are necessary. The purpose of advertising is to convince consumers the product or service is necessary, safe, and effective. Often the advertisement uses testimonials or claims to demonstrate the benefits of using the product. Testimonials are people's personal reports about their positive experiences with a product.

Materials: Health-care product cards (Fig. 7-3), poster boards, crayons, videotaping equipment

Initiation: Write "testimonials" and "claims" on the chalkboard. Ask students to define these terms. Divide students into teams. Give each team a poster board and a health-care product card.

Activity: Have each team invent a type of health care product that matches the product identified on their team's card. They need to give the product an appealing name, price the product, and write an advertisement that will convince others to purchase it. They may want to write a "jingle" to use in their ad. After they develop the product and its advertisement, they are to present their ad to the rest of the class. Videotape "commercials," if it ispossible. Review videotaped commercials for the class to enjoy and evaluate.

Closure: Ask students, "Did any of the ads convince you to try the product? Which advertising features make products appealing?"

CONSUMER HEALTH
INTERMEDIATE LEVEL

Objective: **Interprets information provided on health product labels.**

Level: Grades 4 and 5

Title: *Looking at Labels*

Integration: Comparison, analysis

Vocabulary: None

Content
Generalization: Food packaging labels provide information about the ingredients used in the formulation of the product. Ingredients are listed in descending order by weight. For example, if the first ingredient is water, that means that the product has more water, by weight, than other ingredients. This information is useful when comparing similar products and for those with food allergies. People with certain food allergies can check labels to avoid possible allergic reactions to any ingredient.

Materials: Food packages (various brands of margarine, soups, juices, cereals, and snack items) Handout (Fig. 7- 4) Looking at Labels

Initiation: Arrange food packages where they are visible to students. Have students choose a partner. Write "ingredients" on the chalkboard.

Activity: Give students at least two similar product packages to compare. Ask students to locate the list of ingredients. Have each student complete the handout.

Closure: Ask students to explain the usefulness of ingredient labeling.

CONSUMER HEALTH
INTERMEDIATE LEVEL

Objective:	**Interprets information provided on health product labels.**
Level:	Grade 6
Title:	*Label Fables*
Integration:	Math, comparison, analysis
Vocabulary:	None
Content Generalization:	Food packaging labels provide information about the ingredients used in the formulation of the product. Consumers interested in avoiding too much fat can be misled by some information on labels. Often the product is promoted as a low-fat or "light" product. However, manufacturers may be referring to the percentage of the product recipe (by volume) that is fat, not the percentage of Calories that are fat.
Materials:	Food packages promoted as low-fat, "lite," or fat-reduced (examples include hotdogs, cheeses, margarines, and luncheon meats) Handout (Fig. 7-5) Label Fables
Initiation:	Arrange food packages where they are visible to students. Have students choose a partner. Review how to use labels to determine the number of Calories from fat in each serving. Each gram of fat contributes 9 Calories. Multiply the total number of grams of fat times 9 to determine the number of fat Calories in each serving. To determine the percentage of total Calories from fat, take the number of fat Calories and divide it by the total number of Calories. This number will be a decimal. Multiply by 100 to obtain the percentage.
Activity:	Give students at least two similar product packages to compare. Ask students to locate the nutrient labels. Have each student complete the handout.
Closure:	Ask students to explain the usefulness of nutrient labeling when analyzing claims such as "fat-reduced."

CONSUMER HEALTH
INTERMEDIATE LEVEL

Objective:	**Interprets information provided on health product labels.**
Level:	Grade 5 and 6
Title:	*Brand vs. Generic*
Integration:	Comparison, analysis
Vocabulary:	Brand name, generic
Content	
Generalization:	Advertisers of health-care products offer consumers the promise of becoming more attractive or healthy by using a particular product. People may choose to buy a product based on emotions rather than need. For example, many advertisers sell a particular image to the consumer, often associating the product with a hero. The most attractively packaged and heavily advertised products ("brand" names) usually cost more than simple "generic" products. Furthermore, other similar but less expensive products may be just as effective as the more costly items. Packaging labels provide information about the materials used in the formulation of the product. Ingredients are listed in descending order by weight. For example, if the first ingredient is water, that means that the product has more water, by weight, than other ingredients.
Materials:	Handout (Fig 7-6) Brand Name vs. Generic. Letter explaining project to parents.
Initiation:	Have students obtain parental approval and assistance with this project. Ask students to explain how can they tell what kinds of materials are used to make a health-care product, such as shampoo, hand lotion, soaps, or toothpastes. Ask, "Why do you buy a particular product, such as shampoo?"
Activity:	Give each student a handout. Ask them to go to a store that sells health-care products and choose one, such as shampoo. Students are to complete the product questionnaire and return it within 3 days.
Closure:	Ask, "What did you learn about the health care product you chose to investigate." "Are there many different types from which to choose?" "How helpful is the information on the label?"

91

CONSUMER HEALTH
INTERMEDIATE LEVEL

Objective: **Lists sources of reliable health information and services.**
Level: Grade 6
Title: *Where's the Expert?*
Integration: Language arts, analysis
Vocabulary: Expertise
Content
Generalization: There are many unreliable sources of information in communities including popular books found in bookstores and public libraries, promoters of health food products, and so-called health "experts" who are guests on radio/TV "talk" shows. Anyone can say anything about health; the information does not have to be true. First Amendment rights guarantee freedom of speech; therefore it is often the consumer's responsibility to analyze carefully what they read or hear about health. Reliable sources include health educators and medical professionals including doctors, dentists, and hospital dietitians. Health departments often employ health educators, too.
Materials: None
Initiation: Write the word "expertise" on the chalkboard. Ask students to define the term. Ask, "Who would you ask for legal advice?" (The answer is a lawyer.) "Who would you ask to electrically wire a new house?" (The answer is an electrician.) These individuals have *expertise*. "Who do you ask for nutrition advice?" "Would you read a book written by someone with no obvious credentials?" "Would you ask a clerk in a health food store?" "How can you tell if health advice that you are given is accurate information?" "Who has the *expertise*?"
Activity: Assign students the task of locating a popular health book in the public library. They are to read the book and try to locate passages where they believe the information is questionable or where the author makes claims about a disease, a particular treatment, or a cure. If they can't locate a book, they can visit a local health food store and locate a product that has health claims associated with it. Often health food stores provide free promotional literature about products. They can take a copy of a product's promotional literature and note the product's label information including any health claims. Have them decide who would have the expertise in their community to be able to help them analyze the information for reliability. They are to contact the expert and ask for their help in determining the reliability of the information in question.
Closure: Ask, "Where do you go or who do you ask for reliable health information?"

CONSUMER HEALTH
INTERMEDIATE LEVEL

Objective: **Describes advertising appeal of foods and medications used by children.**

Level: Grades 5 and 6

Title: *Aisle Appeal*

Integration: Math, analysis

Content Generalization: Food products are packaged and marketed to be as appealing as possible to consumers. For example, many of the healthier cereal products are difficult to reach being stacked on higher shelves; those highly sweetened varieties are sold within arms' reach of children. Candy and chewing gum are also sold in check-out lines where children are more likely to hassle parents into making unplanned, unwanted, and unnecessary purchases.

Materials: Handout (Fig. 7-7) Aisle Appeal, empty cereal boxes including high fiber and high sugar varieties

Initiation: Variety of empty cereal boxes. Ask children to decide which boxes are more appealing. Ask "What characteristics of the box appeal to you?" Distribute handout.

Activity: Children are to accompany parents on a trip to the grocery store to complete the questions noted on the handout.

Closure: Ask children, "What did you learn about the way products are marketed in stores to ensure sales?"

CONSUMER HEALTH
INTERMEDIATE LEVEL

Objective: **Describes advertising appeal of foods and medications used by children.**

Level: Grades 5 and 6

Title: *Comic Appeal*

Integration: Analysis

Vocabulary: Supplements

Content Generalization: Food products are packaged and marketed to be as appealing as possible to consumers. Vitamin and mineral supplements are made more appealing to children by having comic character shapes, attractive colors, and sweet tastes. Parents give these to their children, telling them "it's good for you." Unfortunately, every year a number of children poison themselves by eating too many of these supplements.

Materials: Handout (Fig. 7-8) Comic Appeal

Initiation: Ask children if any of them take vitamin/mineral supplements. Which brands do they take? Distribute handout.

Activity: Children are to accompany parents on a trip to the grocery store, pharmacy, or other store where children's nutrient supplements are sold. They are to locate the part of the store where vitamin/mineral supplements are displayed and answer the questions on the handout.

Closure: Ask children, "What did you learn about how children's vitamin/mineral supplements are marketed in stores to ensure sales?"

CONSUMER HEALTH
INTERMEDIATE LEVEL

Objective: **Differentiates between quackery and licensed health care.**
Level: Grade 6
Title: *The Great Debate*
Integration: Science, language arts, analysis
Vocabulary: Quackery, alternative treatment
Content
Generalization: A quack is an unqualified individual who poses as a health expert. Quacks often promote ideas and treatments that are not based upon scientifically held principles. For example, alternative medicine recommends treatments or cures that are not considered to be effective by conventional medical practitioners. Many forms of health quackery are harmless. However, quackery can be costly, hold out the promise of a cure when none exists, and delay the use of a known, effective form of treatment.
Materials: None
Initiation: Write "quackery" on the chalkboard. Ask students to define the term. Divide the class into two teams. One team will represent the medical establishment and consist of doctors, dietitians and nurses. The other team consists of health quacks. The quackery team invents a health-care product or a treatment for a disease that has miraculous value. They are to design a marketing plan, including advertisements, for the product. The quackery team shares their marketing information with the medical establishment team. The medical team reviews the marketing information and determines how the information can be considered unreliable. Both groups spend several days planning for a debate. Each team chooses a panel of three debaters to represent their team's position.
Activity: Set up six chairs for the debate. Invite another class of students in to watch the debate. Give the quackery team 5 minutes to present their product or treatment and describe its benefits. After their presentation, give the medical expert team a 5-minute opportunity to support or rebut the quackery team's claims. Allow each team one additional 5- minute session to convince the audience that their position is correct. Ask the audience to decide which team presented the best case for or against the product or treatment. What made their argument so convincing?
Closure: Ask students, "What questions can you ask to determine if the health care or advice you are receiving is from qualified sources?"

CONSUMER HEALTH
MIDDLE SCHOOL LEVEL

Objective:	**Analyzes methods used to promote health products and services.**
Level:	Grades 7 and 8
Title:	*Ad Fads*
Integration:	Social studies, language arts, analysis
Vocabulary:	None
Content Generalization:	Advertisers of health-care products offer consumers the promise of becoming more attractive by or healthy if they use a particular product. People often choose to buy a product based on emotions rather than need. For example, many advertisers sell a particular image to the consumer, often associating the product with a hero. The most attractively packaged and heavily advertised products ("brand" names) usually cost more than simple "generic" products. Furthermore, other similar but less expensive products may be just as effective as the more costly items.
Materials:	Handout (Fig. 7-9) Ad Fads
Initiation:	Ask students, "Which brands of clothing or shoes are the best?" "Which stores carry the best products?" "How do they feel about wearing clothing with particular labels on them?" "Which labels are popular now?" "Are these items higher quality that similar items manufactured by less trendy companies?"
Activity:	Ask students to look through magazines at home or in the library to find advertisements for alcoholic beverages or tobacco products. Have them make a copy of the advertisement to attach to their handout. (They are to attach a copy and not the actual ad; they are not to tear ads out of library magazines.) Students are to complete and turn in the handout.
Closure:	Ask students, "What makes advertising appeal to you?"

CONSUMER HEALTH
MIDDLE SCHOOL LEVEL

Objective: **Compares scientific and faddish bases for choices among health products.**

Level: Grades 7 and 8

Title: *How Science Works*

Integration: Science, anecdote, comparison

Vocabulary: Fad, anecdote, controls, experiment, placebo

Content Generalization: People may report that some practice or product is beneficial to health. These personal reports are called anecdotes. The practice or product may become a fad, something that is fashionable for a period of time. For example, some people might report that when they take large, daily doses of vitamin C, they have fewer colds. Anecdotes are interesting, but there is no factual evidence that indicates the product or practice actually contributed to the improved state of health. Scientifically controlled experimentation can be useful in determining the facts, including true benefits of a product or practice. Science often seeks to answer questions or uncover facts by controlled experimentation. In a scientifically controlled study of vitamin C and cold prevention, a large group of people could be used; the group is divided in half. One group receives a dose of vitamin C daily (the experimental group), the other receives a placebo instead of the vitamin (the control group). Placebos look and taste like the vitamin but have no effect on the body. Placebos are used to prevent subjects from determining to which group they have been assigned. Both groups make no other changes in their lives except to keep records of the number of colds they have over the study time period. At the end of the recording time period, the number of colds reported in both groups is analyzed. If the vitamin C group has far fewer colds than the placebo group, the researchers may conclude that vitamin C may have some cold prevention benefits. If it does not, they could conclude that vitamin C may have the effect at higher doses than used in this study and they would repeat the study using higher doses. Or, they may just conclude that the practice is a useless health fad.

Materials: Handout (Fig. 7-10) Designing a Study

Initiation: Write the word "anecdote" on the chalkboard. Ask students if they know the meaning of this word. Ask students if they have ever heard any anecdotes about the healthful or healing properties of some product. Explain the features of a scientifically designed study to students. Divide students into teams of about five students.

Activity: Give each team of students the handout. Explain that they are to follow the guidelines for designing a scientific study. Ask each team to present their experimental design to the class.

Closure: Ask students what may happen when a fad is scientifically tested.

CONSUMER HEALTH
MIDDLE SCHOOL LEVEL

Objective: **Compares scientific and faddish bases for choices among health products.**

Level: Grades 7 and 8

Title: *The Claim Game*

Integration: Science, analysis

Vocabulary: None

Content Generalization: Many health-care products and services use promotional claims. These claims are general statements that may be difficult to prove or verify. For example, consider the statement, "Nine out of ten doctors trust Conitrol." Does this mean that 90% of the medical doctors polled or 9 of the 10 Ph.D.s who work for the product's manufacturer?

Materials: Handout (Fig. 7- 11) The Claim Game, two sample ads from a magazine or newspaper with typical claims concerning the product's effectiveness. Videotaped commercials are also effective.

Initiation: Display one ad where it is visible. Ask students what they think about the claim. Ask students to find a partner. Give each pair a handout to complete.

Activity: Students are to take about 30 minutes to analyze the claims. Ask students to review each claim.

Closure: Display the second ad. Ask students to analyze this ad for misleading claims.

CONSUMER HEALTH
MIDDLE SCHOOL LEVEL

Objective:	**Describes the function of consumer-protection agencies.**
Level:	Grades 7 and 8
Title:	*Agencies That Work*
Integration:	Social studies
Vocabulary:	FDA, agencies
Content Generalization:	The government has established agencies to protect the consumer and to see that federal laws are being followed. The Food and Drug Administration (FDA) is a branch of the U.S. Public Health Service. The agency's primary function is to protect consumers from unsafe or ineffective health-care products including hazardous foods, cosmetics, medications, and medical devices.
Materials:	Invitation to local FDA official.
Initiation:	Write "Food and Drug Administration (FDA)" on the chalkboard.
Activity:	Have the guest spend about 30 minutes explaining the consumer protection functions of the FDA and answering students' questions.
Closure:	Ask students what they think would happen if there were no consumer protection agencies like the FDA.

CONSUMER HEALTH
MIDDLE SCHOOL LEVEL

Objective: **Identifies criteria for the selection of a qualified health advisor.**

Level: Grades 6 and 7

Title: *Making Choices*

Integration: Social studies, analysis

Vocabulary: Medical practitioner

Content Generalization: Qualified health advisors are prepared at educational facilities that are recognized, often by a national or state accrediting group, as offering high quality and up-to-date training. The training for these professions is often demanding and rigorous. Many medical specialties require members to undergo continuing educational training to maintain their level of knowledge and skill. Choosing the best medical practitioner may involve asking others to recommend someone, checking the practitioner's credentials, and interviewing the prospective medical specialist to determine if one will be comfortable with the choice. Developing a sense of trust and rapport between practitioner and client is important.

Materials: Handout (7-12) Choosing a Health Advisor

Initiation: Ask students how they feel about any of their medical practitioners, such as a doctor or dentist. What do they like or dislike about the practitioner? Give students the handout. Explain that they will need to interview a parent or grandparent to complete the assignment.

Activity: Students conduct the adult interview and complete the handout.

Closure: Ask students, "Which factors seem to be the most important to consider?"

AVOIDING DRUG MISUSE
Student Objectives

Primary Level K-3 Student:

1. Explains reasons for avoiding use of controlled drugs or unknown substances.
2. Explains reasons why many people avoid using any drugs, including tobacco and alcohol.
3. Demonstrates effective ways of refusing offers of drugs.

Intermediate Level 4-5/6 Student:

1. Analyzes reasons why some people abuse drugs.
2. Explains why we have laws controlling use of drugs.
3. Evaluates the effectiveness of problem-solving skills in choosing alternatives to drug use.

Middle School Level 6/7-8 Student:

1. Predicts effects of drugs on physical, mental, and social functioning.
2. Analyzes factors motivating individuals to avoid or abuse drugs.
3. Interprets the significance of peer pressure on decisions regarding drug use.

AVOIDING DRUG MISUSE
PRIMARY LEVEL

Objective: **Explains reasons for avoiding use of controlled drugs or unknown substances.**

Level: Grade 3

Title: *I Have a Dream*

Integration: Language arts, art

Vocabulary: Goals, substance abuse, marijuana, crack, cocaine, tobacco, alcohol

Content Generalization: Thinking about the future and setting goals are important activities for youngsters. Youngsters can determine how drug abuse interferes with their ability to achieve goals. Substance abuse has negative effects on physical health and social relationships. Substance abuse convictions can damage one's ability to find employment as well.

Materials: I Have a Dream Bulletin Board, paper, crayons

Initiation: Prepare a plain bulletin board with the title "I Have A Dream." Ask children if they ever dream about what they would like to be doing in the future. Ask them to describe their future situations. Ask, "What do you think will happen to your future if you take drugs like cocaine or alcohol?" Tell children not to name anyone, but ask if they know someone who drinks too much alcohol, smokes cigarettes or uses other tobacco products, or abuses illegal drugs like marijuana, crack, or LSD. Can they describe some of the effects this abuse has had on these people, their family, and friends? Ask, "What happens when people who drink alcohol or smoke marijuana try to drive?" "What can happen to people who may be on the same road at the same time as the substance abuser?" "What is wrong with abusing controlled drugs or unknown substances that affect the body?" "What are other ways substance abuse affects your life?"

Activity: Have children think about what they want to be doing 5 years from now. Have them draw a picture of themselves as drug-free individuals. Post pictures on the bulletin board.

Closure: Ask children to think about what their picture would look like if they were *abusing* a controlled substance or unknown drug 5 years from now. Ask, "What would be different about your picture?"

AVOIDING DRUG MISUSE
PRIMARY LEVEL

Objective:	**Explains reasons why many people avoid using any drugs, including tobacco and alcohol.**
Level:	Grade 3
Title:	*Living Free*
Integration:	Social studies, analysis
Vocabulary:	Substance abuse, addiction/dependence, marijuana, crack, cocaine, tobacco, alcohol
Content Generalization:	Some people choose not to use mind-altering substances because of religious reasons, health reasons, or their occupations. Others may have lived with an addicted or dependent person and do not want to follow their example. These people find drug-free alternatives to keep their minds stimulated. They know that substance abuse is not a solution to their problems.
Materials:	None
Initiation:	Ask students to identify mind-altering substances. They should mention alcohol, tobacco, crack, cocaine, LSD, glues, and marijuana. Ask students if they know someone who does **not** use controlled or unknown substances to alter their minds.
Activity:	Ask students to interview a person over the age 15 who does not use mind-altering drugs. Children are to explore reasons why the individual chose to be drug-free. Have students write a one page biography of their drug-free person that includes their reasons for living drug-free.
Closure:	Ask students the reasons people gave for choosing to be drug-free. List their reasons on the chalkboard.

AVOIDING DRUG MISUSE
PRIMARY LEVEL

Objective: **Demonstrates effective ways of refusing offers of drugs.**

Level: Grade 3

Title: *Saying Nope to Dopes Without Hope*

Integration: Language arts

Vocabulary: Peer pressure, skit

Content Generalization: Children need to practice refusal skills to be able to respond assertively when situations involving use of a dangerous substance occur. Role-playing is an effective and enjoyable way to teach refusal skills.

Materials: Props for role-play skits

Initiation: Ask children to think of situations in which peers apply pressure. It may be to play a particular game, watch a TV program, or try a drug such as tobacco, marijuana, or alcohol. Divide class into teams of six students.

Activity: Each team is to write a brief skit about characters who are in situations in which drug experimentation is occurring. Each situation should have an individual who is applying the peer pressure and one who is refusing. If they need any props, they should try to make them from materials available. Each student team acts out their skit. After each skit, ask students to critique the skit. How effective were the refusal skills used in each of the situations presented?

Closure: Ask students to identify effective peer pressure refusal techniques.

AVOIDING DRUG MISUSE
INTERMEDIATE LEVEL

Objective: **Analyzes reasons why some people abuse drugs.**

Level: Grade 5

Title: *Why Some Choose to Abuse*

Integration: Analysis

Vocabulary: None

Content Generalization: People who are long-term substance abusers often suffer from low self-esteem. They may see their lives as hopeless and painful and believe that substance abuse provides an escape from their negative feelings.

Materials: None

Initiation: Ask children, "Why do you think people abuse drugs?"

Activity: Invite a guest speaker from a hospital or community-based mental health center to present a 30 minute description of reasons why people become addicted to mind-altering substances. Have students ask the guest about which young people may be more likely to become addicted. Can you predict who is likely to become dependent on drugs?

Closure: Ask children to write a one-page essay, entitled "Why Some Choose to Abuse." The essays can be read to the class or posted on a bulletin board.

AVOIDING DRUG MISUSE
INTERMEDIATE LEVEL

Objective:	**Analyzes reasons why some people abuse drugs.**
Level:	Grade 4
Title:	*Abuse Clues*
Integration:	Social studies, analysis
Vocabulary:	Mind-altering, peer pressure
Content Generalization:	People who are long-term substance abusers often suffer from low self-esteem. They may see their lives as hopeless and painful, and believe that substance abuse provides an escape from their negative feelings. Reasons often given for youthful drug experimentation include: being curious, bored, "stressed-out," or afraid to lose friends. Other youngsters want to look "cool," take risks, control their weight, or feel mature.
Materials:	None
Initiation:	Divide children into teams of three students. Write "drug abuse" on the chalkboard.
Activity:	While working in teams, children brainstorm reasons why young people decide to experiment with or abuse mind-altering drugs. Each team compiles a list of possible reasons. Ask one child from each team to write their list of reasons on the chalkboard. Determine which team thought of the most possible reasons. Were any reasons mentioned by more than one team?
Closure:	Ask students to rank the reasons for drug experimentation in order from most likely to least likely reasons.

AVOIDING DRUG MISUSE
INTERMEDIATE LEVEL

Objective:	**Explains why we have laws controlling the use of drugs.**
Level:	Grade 6
Title:	*Keeping Drugs Under Control*
Integration:	Social studies
Vocabulary:	Regulation, toxic
Content Generalization:	Regulating drug use through laws is believed to be for the public good. Drug abuse has negative effects on health, job functioning, and interpersonal relationships. It also contributes to our nation's crime problem.
Materials:	None
Initiation:	Write "Drug Enforcement Administration" on the chalkboard. Ask students why are regulations controlling the production, sale, and possession of toxic drugs necessary?
Activity:	Invite a guest speaker, an agent of the Drug Enforcement Administration or local law enforcement agency representative, to describe his or her job. Why are these kinds of law enforcement jobs necessary? Some want to change the laws so that the use of many illegal drugs would be permitted. What does the drug law enforcement representative think would happen if these substances were legalized?
Closure:	Ask students to write a one-page essay on the reasons why they think the use of mind-altering substances should remain controlled or illegal.

AVOIDING DRUG MISUSE
INTERMEDIATE LEVEL

Objective:	**Evaluates the effectiveness of problem-solving skills in choosing alternatives to drug use.**
Level:	Grades 5 and 6
Title:	*People Solve Problems, Not Drugs*
Integration:	Social studies, analysis
Vocabulary:	Pros, cons
Content Generalization:	Problem-solving skills need to be learned and practiced. Youngsters need to realize that drug abuse does not solve problems, it creates them. Every problem has at least one solution. The challenge is having individuals develop the creative problem-solving skills that enable them to find effective and healthy solutions.
Materials:	Handout (Fig 8-1) Pros and Cons
Initiation:	Write "pros" and "cons" on the chalkboard. Ask students to describe a situation in which they had to make a choice. How do you make choices? Explain that one way is to determine each of the possible choices and weigh what would be benefits (pros) and risks (cons) of each choice. Ask students to work in pairs.
Activity:	Give each pair of students a handout and about 15 minutes to complete the assignment.
Closure:	Ask students why using drugs is not an effective way to deal with life's problems.

AVOIDING DRUG MISUSE
MIDDLE SCHOOL LEVEL

Objective: **Predicts the effect of drugs on physical, mental, and social functioning.**

Level: Grades 6 through 8

Title: *Liver Business*

Integration: Science, prediction

Vocabulary: Detoxification, alcohol, molecules, enzymes

Content Generalization: The liver is an extremely important organ. One of its many functions is to detoxify dangerous drugs. It does this if it has the necessary enzymes to take apart the dangerous chemicals and convert them to less harmful substances. The liver can detoxify only a set amount of the toxic chemical within a period of time. For example, when an individual drinks a small amount of alcohol, he or she may not become drunk because the liver is able to convert the alcohol molecule to safer substances. However, if the individual drinks too much alcohol at one time, the liver cannot speed up its rate of detoxification. The high levels of alcohol remain in the blood and cause drunkenness and damage to the body.

Materials: 40 large plastic infant toys that snap together, box

Initiation: Write "liver" and "enzymes" on the chalkboard. Explain that enzymes are needed to change a toxic chemical, such as alcohol, to less harmful substances.

Activity: Have a child sit on the floor and identify this place as the liver. The child represents the liver's alcohol-destroying enzyme. Explain that each two-piece plastic snap toy represents one molecule of the chemical alcohol. The liver enzyme's job is to break apart the alcohol so that it is no longer harmful. Have another child stand in front of the liver and toss one plastic toy (two plastic pieces snapped together) at the enzyme. The enzyme takes the toy, unsnaps it into two pieces, and tosses the pieces into the box. Have them repeat this three times. Ask the "tossing" child to take a handful of the toys and empty them on top of the enzyme. The enzyme continues unsnapping the toys but becomes overwhelmed with the amount of work.

Closure: Ask students why the enzyme could not unsnap all of the alcohol that was dumped into the liver. Ask students to predict what happens when a person drinks too much alcohol at one time.

AVOIDING DRUG MISUSE
MIDDLE SCHOOL LEVEL

Objective: **Predicts the effect of drugs on physical, mental, and social functioning.**

Level: Grades 6 and 7

Title: *Choking with Smoking*

Integration: Science

Vocabulary: Tar, nicotine

Content Generalization: Tobacco smoke contains hundreds of chemicals. Many of these are known to cause cancer and damage arteries, leading to cardiovascular diseases. Tar is a sticky substance that contains several cancer-causing agents. People cannot see how their bodies are damaged by years of smoking. Often the first signs of serious health problems occur when cancers or cardiovascular diseases are well-established and beyond a cure.

Materials: Mechanical smoking device with a white cloth that traps tar, available from Lung Association or a supplier of health education products; cigarette; matches

Initiation: Ask students if they know someone who smokes cigarettes. What do they smell like?

Activity: Using the mechanical smoker, smoke the cigarette. Remove the cloth and show students how one cigarette yellowed the cloth. Ask students if they know what caused the yellow discoloration (tar).

Closure: Ask students to predict what happens to lungs of smokers over many years of smoking.

AVOIDING DRUG MISUSE
MIDDLE SCHOOL LEVEL

Objective: **Predicts effects of drugs on physical, mental, and social functioning.**

Level: Grade 6

Title: *Drugs Destroy Destinies*

Integration: Social studies, language arts, prediction

Vocabulary: Dependence, addiction, detoxification

Content Generalization: Drug abuse has negative effects on health, job functioning, families, and interpersonal relationships. It also contributes to our nation's crime problem. Many people are able to disengage themselves from the addiction. Their insights can be useful in helping youngsters see the damaging effects of substance abuse.

Materials: Invitation to a recovered alcoholic or other drug addict. Contact local hospitals and drug education agencies for names of people who like to speak to youngsters about the hazards associated with substance abuse.

Initiation: Ask children to prepare questions about substance abuse for the guest speaker. Arrange chairs in a circle around the guest speaker.

Activity: Have the guest speaker spend 30 minutes talking about their former addicted lifestyle. The remaining time should be allotted for student questions.

Closure: Ask youngsters to write a two-page science-fiction essay about how their life changed the day they became addicted to a drug. Have children write thank-you notes and send them to the guest speaker.

AVOIDING DRUG MISUSE
MIDDLE SCHOOL LEVEL

Objective:	**Analyzes factors motivating individuals to avoid or abuse drugs.**
Level:	Grades 7 and 8
Title:	*Freedom From Drugs*
Integration:	Language arts, interpersonal, analysis
Vocabulary:	None
Content Generalization:	Some people are motivated to avoid using mind-altering substances because of religious reasons, health concerns, or their occupations. Others may have lived with an addicted or dependent person and do not want to follow their example. These people find drug-free alternatives to keep their minds stimulated. They know that substance abuse is not a solution to their problems.
Materials:	None
Initiation:	Ask students if they know someone who does not use mind-altering drugs.
Activity:	Students are to identify and interview a person who does not use mind-altering drugs. It can be someone who has recovered from a drug addiction. After the interview, students determine factors that are important in motivating people to avoid substance abuse.
Closure:	Students submit a written analysis of the factors that influenced the person to avoid substance abuse.

AVOIDING DRUG MISUSE
MIDDLE SCHOOL LEVEL

Objective:	**Interprets the significance of peer pressure on decisions regarding drug use.**
Level:	Grade 7
Title:	*The Power of Peer Pressure*
Integration:	Language arts
Vocabulary:	Peer pressure
Content Generalization:	Peer pressure influences decisions youngsters make concerning health. Important skills include being able to recognize when peer pressure occurs and analyze the situation to avoid negative outcomes.
Materials:	Props as needed
Initiation:	Announce that the class will write a play about how youngsters can recognize peer pressure and refuse alcohol. This play will be presented to a class of sixth graders. Divide students into teams of writers, actors, and set "designers." The first team writes the script and directs the team of actors. The designer team prepares or collects the play's props.
Activity:	Students are given 2 days to write a script for the play. Actors are assigned their roles and given an opportunity to practice in front of the class. After several rehearsals, invite a sixth grade class into the classroom to watch the play.
Closure:	Ask students to determine how much peer pressure influences young peoples' decision-making processes, especially decisions involving drug experimentation.

ENVIRONMENTAL HEALTH
Student Objectives

Primary Level K-3 Student:

1. Identifies the sources of environmental (air, land, and water) pollution.
2. Names actions that conserve natural resources.
3. Describes ways to work with others to help provide a healthful environment.

Intermediate Level 4-5/6 Student:

1. Explains how improving the environment can enhance physical, social, and mental health.
2. Identifies causes and preventives against environmental pollution.

Middle School Level 6/7-8 Student:

1. Analyzes ways individuals and communities can promote a healthful and safe environment.
2. Evaluates the effects of community groups and agencies in improving and protecting the environment.

ENVIRONMENTAL HEALTH
PRIMARY LEVEL

Objective: **Identifies the sources of environmental (air, land, and water) pollution.**

Level: Grade 3

Title: *Paper, Paper, Everywhere*

Integration: Science, language arts

Vocabulary: Pollution, landfill, environment, resources

Content Generalization: The typical American family throws out almost 100 pounds of trash each week. About one-half of the paper produced in the U.S. is used as packaging material that is thrown out. Also "junk mail," often unwanted and unread, is thrown out. Excess use of paper products reduces an important environmental resource, trees. Furthermore this paper waste is filling up our landfills.

Materials: Bag of 1 week's collection of junk mail, envelopes, permission letter from parents

Initiation: Send a letter to the parents explaining the objective of the activity. Ask for their permission to send a letter to a direct marketing group that will remove their names from mailing lists. If the parent does not approve, the child can still write a letter, but do not mail it with the others. Write "pollution" on the chalkboard. Ask children to define the term. Ask if their parents consider junk mail a form of pollution. Show children the kinds of unwanted mail that was received in 1 week.

Activity: Ask children to return the parental permission letter. Children are to compose and write a letter to: Mail Preference Service, PO Box 9008, Farmingdale, NY, 11735-9008. The letter should request to have their parents' names removed from the bulk mailing lists of many of the larger companies. It helps to include a mailing label removed from a piece of the family's unwanted mail.

Children are to take the letter home for parents to read and sign. Ask parents to provide a sample mailing label and a stamp. Children learn to address the envelope and mail the letter.

Closure: Ask children, "What is the problem with "junk mail?"

ENVIRONMENTAL HEALTH
PRIMARY LEVEL

Objective:	**Identifies the sources of environmental (air, land, and water) pollution.**
Level:	Grade 3
Title:	*Fantastic Plastic*
Integration:	Science
Vocabulary:	Pollution, plastic, environment, recycle
Content Generalization:	Plastic soda bottles and milk cartons are recyclable. Recycled plastics are used to make helmets, building material, and even carpeting.
Materials:	Samples of plastic recyclable materials (soda bottles, coffee can lids, plastic shopping bags, plastic rings from beverage six-packs, plastic wrap, and milk cartons)
Initiation:	Place the plastic recyclables where they are visible. Ask children, "What do these things have in common?" Ask, "How many of your families recycle plastic waste?"
Activity:	Ask children to keep a list of all of the plastic waste that their household produces in 1 week. After 1 week, ask children to describe the kinds and amounts of plastic waste thrown out or recycled at their house. Did the amount of plastic waste have any relationship to the number of people in each household?
Closure:	Ask children to think of ways they can reuse plastic material at home.

ENVIRONMENTAL HEALTH
PRIMARY LEVEL

Objective: **Identifies the sources of environmental (air, land, and water) pollution**

Level: Grade 3

Title: *Find the Pollutant*

Integration: Science

Vocabulary: Pesticide, pollution, pollutant

Content Generalization: Land, air, and water pollution threaten the quality of our environment. Many pollutants are created by humans, including pesticides, packaging materials, human wastes, food wastes, items that are no longer useful, and paper used for communication. Children can learn to identify some of the more familiar pollutants and become more aware of pollution's threat to their environment.

Materials: Handout (Fig. 9-1) Find the Pollutant. Key to Find the Pollutant (Fig. 9-2)

Initiation: Write the terms "pesticide," "pollution," and "pollutant" on the chalkboard. Ask children if they know what these words mean.

Activity: Ask children to pair up with another student. Give each pair a copy of the handout. They will need about 10-15 minutes to try to identify all of the sources of pollution in the handout.

Closure: Ask each team to identify sources of pollution shown in the handout. Identify those sources that are not identified by the students.

ENVIRONMENTAL HEALTH
PRIMARY LEVEL

Objective:	**Names actions that conserve natural resources.**
Level:	Grade 3
Title:	*Recycle That Paper!*
Integration:	Science, art
Vocabulary:	Recycle
Content	
Generalization:	Many man-made materials can be recycled or converted to another function. Paper is among the easiest material to recycle. It is estimated that if everyone recycled just 10% of their newspaper waste, about 25 million trees could be saved each year.
Materials:	Cardboard boxes, recycle paper signs. Check with the administration and the district's waste disposal company about the feasibility of establishing a paper recycling program. Follow their guidelines concerning the kinds of paper that can be accepted.
Initiation:	Ask children what living thing is used to make paper. Ask them to identify what kinds of products use paper. Explain to children that the use of so much paper, including disposable diapers, junk mail, school ditto handouts, and newsprint, creates pollution. Ask, "How are many communities trying to deal with the problem of too much paper waste?" The answer is recycling programs.
Activity:	Children are to take cardboard boxes and convert them into paper recycling containers for classrooms. They can decorate the boxes and make signs that identify them for paper recycling. Ask for a student volunteer to contact the district's waste disposal company to determine paper recycling guidelines. This information will have to be distributed to all of the classrooms participating in the paper recycling program. Children will have to make weekly "pick-ups" at the participating classrooms to collect the paper recycling boxes and empty them into the larger paper collection bins provided by company that has agreed to collect the recyclable paper.
Closure:	Ask children, "What are the benefits of recycling paper?"

ENVIRONMENTAL HEALTH
PRIMARY LEVEL

Objective: **Names actions that conserve natural resources.**

Level: Grade 3

Title: *Recycling Works*

Integration: Science

Vocabulary: Recycling

Content Generalization: Many man-made materials can be recycled or converted to another function. Paper is among the easiest material to recycle. Many larger communities have recycling centers that also collect glass, aluminum, and plastics. With a little creativity, many plastic items and metal cans can be turned into useful items for home use. For example, soup cans can be converted into crayon or pencil holders. Plastic margarine tubs can be used to store beads, embroidery thread, or leftover foods.

Materials: Plastic milk cartons, thin wood doweling, string, scissors. Fig. 9-3 (Bird feeder and scoop instructions)

Initiation: Have children bring in plastic milk cartons. Ask, "How many of your families recycle household waste products?" "What kinds of materials does your family recycle?" People can recycle items that are thrown out by finding new uses for them.

Activity: Show children a plastic milk carton. Ask them, "What can you make out of a milk carton that can be useful?" Show the class how to make a bird feeder. Or, show children how to make a scoop for removing ashes from a charcoal grill, scooping out kitty litter, or salting icy walkways in winter. Each child makes an object for household use out of their waste milk carton.

Closure: Ask children, "Can you think of ways to recycle soup cans, plastic margarine tubs, or other household plastics that are usually thrown away?"

ENVIRONMENTAL HEALTH
PRIMARY LEVEL

Objective: **Describes ways to work with others to provide a healthful environment.**
Level: Grade 3
Title: *Adopt a Road*
Integration: Social studies
Vocabulary: Litter, environment
Content
Generalization: Litter is garbage that is strewn along roadsides, in vacant lots, and in areas where people live, work, and play. It is an ugly reminder of human thoughtlessness and disregard for the environment. Also, litter may provide a breeding ground for disease-carrying vermin. When children learn to care for a part of their environment by collecting litter, they begin to recognize how littering harms our environment. Perhaps they will be less likely to create litter themselves.
Materials: Gloves, bright orange or red vests, plastic garbage bags
Initiation: Invite classroom parents to help supervise children. **Obtain your administrator's approval** for the activity. Ask children to define "litter" and provide examples.
Activity: Ask parents to help supervise children. Wearing vests and gloves, children pick up litter along the sides of the road by the school or on the playground. Litter is divided into recyclable material or garbage and handled accordingly. This activity may need to be repeated monthly.
Closure: Ask children, "What are other ways we can work together to keep our environment clean and healthy?"

ENVIRONMENTAL HEALTH
INTERMEDIATE LEVEL

Objective:	**Explains how improving the environment can enhance physical, social and mental health.**
Level:	Grades 4 through 6
Title:	*Garden Power*
Integration:	Social studies, language arts
Vocabulary:	None
Content Generalization:	In many urban settings, vacant lots are used as dump sites. These lots are ugly reminders of human thoughtlessness and disregard for the environment. Also, the garbage dumped in these places provides homes for disease-carrying vermin. When children learn to care for a part of their environment by cleaning up these areas and converting them into functional gardens, they take pride in their ability to change and improve a part of their community.
Materials:	Gardening tools, fencing, seeds and seedlings
Initiation:	**Obtain your administrator's approval for the project.** Have children identify an empty lot that is near the school. Children contact community officials to determine if they can use the lot for a garden. Some communities have urban gardening projects. Individuals associated with these projects can be contacted for assistance. Once children have **written** approval from community leaders, they can initiate the project. Children are to compose letters to local hardware stores explaining the project and asking for donations of gardening supplies. Students can also contact the local media to help promote the project. Often with media help, people or companies who will donate supplies are identified.
Activity:	Depending upon the climate and time of year, children clean up a vacant lot and prepare it for a garden. Use of natural fertilizers and pesticides should be encouraged. Children are assigned to plant various flowers, fruits, and vegetables. They weed and care for the garden. When harvested, produce can be eaten by the class or, if approved, sold.
Closure:	Ask children, "How can we improve our health by improving our environment?"

ENVIRONMENTAL HEALTH
INTERMEDIATE LEVEL

Objective:	**Identifies causes of and preventives against environmental pollution.**
Level:	Grades 5 and 6
Title:	*Polluting our Planet*
Integration:	Social studies, language arts
Vocabulary:	Pollution, pollutants
Content	
Generalization:	Land, air, and water pollution threaten the quality of our environment. Many pollutants are created by humans, including pesticides, packaging materials, human wastes, food wastes, items that are no longer useful, and paper used for communication. Environmental disasters create pollution. Some occur locally, such as when a tank car loaded with a hazardous material overturns and spills its load into a stream. Others are major news events, such as the case of the *Exxon Valdez* and the Chernobyl nuclear power plant disasters. Youngsters can explore the reasons behind such disasters and identify ways to avoid future cases of environmental damage.
Materials:	*National Geographic* Magazine articles: Chernobyl- One Year After, page 632, May 1987 Are We Poisoning our Air?, page 502, April 1987 Can We Save This Fragile Earth?, page 858, December 1988 Alaska's Big Spill, page 5, January 1990 Hanging in the Balance, page 2, June1993
Initiation:	Ask students or teachers to bring in copies of these issues. Public libraries often have back issues of *National Geographic* that they will give to school teachers. Using laminated pictures from the *National Geographic* magazines, prepare a bulletin board entitled "Polluting Our Planet." Ask students to identify types of hazardous wastes. Ask if they are aware of any recent accidents that released hazardous waste into the environment.
Activity:	Assign students to work in teams to investigate environmental disasters. Each team is assigned a disaster to research. They are to determine when, where, and how the disaster happened. What can be done to prevent similar disasters from occurring? They will need at least a week to collect information and prepare reports. Reports are to be written as news accounts of the incidents. In a TV news program format, members from each team report on their environmental disaster. They can "interview" public officials, people affected by the disaster, and those responsible.
Closure:	Ask students to write an essay that identifies causes of environmental pollution.

ENVIRONMENTAL HEALTH
MIDDLE SCHOOL LEVEL

Objective: **Analyzes ways individuals and communities can promote a healthful and safe environment.**

Level: Grade 7

Title: *Household Hazards*

Integration: Science

Vocabulary: None

Content Generalization: Many items used in households contain hazardous materials. A hazardous material has the potential to start fires, explode under certain conditions, corrode materials, or poison people or animals. One should not simply throw hazardous household wastes into the garbage or flush them into sewers. These kinds of wastes require special collection and treatment to avoid harming our natural resources.

Materials: Copies of the pamphlet: *Household Hazardous Waste: What you should and shouldn't do*. Available from:
Water Environment Federation
601 Wythe Street
Alexandria, Virginia 22314-1994
Phone: (703) 684-2400

Initiation: Ask students, "What do your parents do to get rid of unwanted household waste, such as paints, varnishes, oven cleaners, insect poisons, or old batteries?" "Do you think they are disposing them in a way that does not pollute?"

Activity: Ask students to identify one potentially hazardous household waste product in their home. They are to investigate how to dispose of this product in an environmentally safe manner.

Closure: Ask students to share the information in the brochure with their parents.

ENVIRONMENTAL HEALTH
MIDDLE SCHOOL LEVEL

Objective: Evaluates the effects of community groups and agencies in improving and protecting the environment.

Level: Grade 8

Title: *Clean Water*

Integration: Science

Vocabulary: Dissolved oxygen, biochemical oxygen demand, effluent, sludge

Content Generalization: Waste water resulting from human use must be treated before being released into waterways. The quality of waste water is measured by factors, such as the biochemical oxygen demand (BOD) and dissolved oxygen. The lower the BOD, the better the effluent (water leaving the treatment plant); the higher the dissolved oxygen, the better the effluent. High quality effluent is released into streams where it does not harm aquatic life. Sludge is the semi-solid material that remains after the water is treated. Sludge is also treated and disposed of according to federal and state regulations. These and other water treatment regulations protect us from waterborne diseases that are prevalent in countries without such high water quality standards.

Materials: None

Initiation: Make arrangements for a field trip to a waste water treatment plant.

Activity: Visit the waste water treatment plant.

Closure: Ask students, "What happens to our quality of life when water becomes contaminated?"

COMMUNITY HEALTH
Student Objectives

Primary Level K-3 Student:

1. Identifies familiar community health workers (health helpers).
2. Explains the functions of various health workers in the community.
3. Lists services provided by community health agencies and organizations.

Intermediate Level 4-5/6 Student:

1. Describes ways community members work together to solve health problems.
2. Identifies functions of interesting career opportunities in the health field.

Middle School Level 6/7-8 Student:

1. Describes community efforts to prevent and control disease.
2. Concludes that individual participation is essential if community health activities are to be successful.

COMMUNITY HEALTH
PRIMARY LEVEL

Objective: **Identifies familiar community health workers (health helpers).**

Level: Grade 1

Title: *Healthy Matches*

Integration: Social studies, reading readiness

Vocabulary: Pharmacist

Content Generalization: Communities offer a wide variety of health services for people. Health services are provided by workers such as dentists, doctors, nurses, pharmacists, and eye doctors. These specially trained individuals can help prevent, detect, and treat diseases, making our lives more enjoyable.

Materials: Handout (Fig. 10-1) Healthy Matches

Initiation: Ask, "How many of you have visited a health care worker in the past month?" Write "eye doctor," "dentist," "doctor," and "pharmacist" on the chalkboard. Ask if any of the children can read these words. What do each of these words mean?

Activity: Have children complete the handout. When the handouts are completed, ask children to explain how they matched the pictures with the words.

Closure: Ask children to name other kinds of health-care workers.

127

COMMUNITY HEALTH
PRIMARY LEVEL

Objective:	**Explains the function of various health workers in the community.**
Level:	Grade 3
Title:	*What if...?*
Integration:	Social studies, language arts, analysis
Vocabulary:	None
Content Generalization:	Communities offer a wide variety of health services for people. Health-care services are provided by workers such as dentists, doctors, nurses, pharmacists, and eye doctors. Police, firefighters, and restaurant inspectors help protect us. These specially trained individuals can help prevent, detect and treat diseases, and keep us safe. Their services help make our lives safer and more enjoyable.
Materials:	None
Initiation:	Invite a firefighter or restaurant inspector in to explain how they play an important role in protecting people.
Activity:	Write the following on the chalkboard: " The day my town had..."
	No doctors
	No nurses
	No eye doctors
	No restaurant inspectors
	No firefighters
	No police
	No pharmacists
	Ask children to choose one of these situations. Each child is to write an essay describing the day their town did not have anyone offering that kind of health-care or protection.
Closure:	Ask for volunteers to read their essays to the rest of the class.

COMMUNITY HEALTH
PRIMARY LEVEL

Objective:	**Lists services provided by community health agencies and organizations.**
Level:	Grade 3
Title:	*Handy Health Helpers*
Integration:	Social studies, analysis
Content Generalization:	Most large communities have health departments or hospitals that provide a variety of health-care services including preventive care, treatment, referrals, and education.
Materials:	Letter to a hospital or health department public relations department to invite an individual who can explain the services of the institution or agency.
Initiation:	Write the name of the hospital or agency represented by the guest speaker. Ask children if they have visited this hospital or health department.
Activity:	Have the guest spend 20 minutes presenting information about the services of their institution or agency. Children are to ask questions about those services.
Closure:	Ask students to identify hospital or health department services that their families are likely to use.

COMMUNITY HEALTH
INTERMEDIATE LEVEL

Objective: **Describes ways community members work together to solve health problems.**

Level: Grade 6

Title: *Mastering Mosquitoes*

Integration: Science, social studies

Vocabulary: Eradication, publicity

Content Generalization: Members from agencies, such as local governments, health departments, hospitals, the news media, and public works departments can work together to solve health problems.

Materials: None

Initiation: Write "public works department officials," "city officials," "news people," "hospital," and "health department workers" on the chalkboard. Describe the following situation to the class: Last summer Fun City experienced more rain than usual. Water collected in old tires, garbage cans, and low-lying areas. Within a few weeks, health department officials began to report an increase in the number of cases of a disease known to be spread by mosquitoes. Now, health department officials have decided that something has to be done to eradicate the insects. They think some publicity from the news media will help educate Fun City's residents. However, city officials are expressing concern about the effect on the city's economy if news of the health problem becomes known. What if the news makes people afraid to vacation in Fun City?

Activity: Ask students to serve as: 1) city officials, 2) health department workers, 3) hospital workers, 4) public works officials, and 5) members of the news media. Divide the classroom into five areas, and direct each team of students to move their seats to that area. Each team considers the mosquito disease problem and decides to take a particular role in dealing with the problem. Give the following instructions to each team:
City officials are concerned about the effects of any negative publicity.
Hospital workers are concerned that they will not be able to treat people.
Health department workers want to educate people about the problem.
Public works officials need the OK to use pesticides to kill the mosquitos and remove trash where the insects breed.
Members of the news media want to report the problem to the public. After determining a strategy for their team, the entire class meets and role-plays their team's position on the health problem. Can they decide on an appropriate course of action?

Closure: Ask students to describe how well they were able to work together as concerned members of a community to achieve goals.

COMMUNITY HEALTH
INTERMEDIATE LEVEL

Objective: Identifies functions of interesting career opportunities in the health field.

Level: Grade 6

Title: *Working for Health*

Integration: Social studies, interpersonal

Vocabulary: Technician

Content Generalization: The health-care field offers a wide variety of interesting and rewarding career opportunities. Many technician positions require 2-year training; physician training involves several years of education and clinical experience.

Materials: None

Initiation: Ask, "How many of you have a parent or grandparent who has a health-related career?" Write their occupations on the chalkboard.

Activity: Ask students to brainstorm health careers that were not mentioned. Students are to choose a health career to explore. As part of the exploration, they are to interview an individual in that particular field. They are to design the interview questions to determine why the person chose that health-care occupation and what educational preparation was necessary.

Closure: Ask, "Now that you have explored a particular health career, do you still think it would be a good choice for your future?" Why?

COMMUNITY HEALTH
MIDDLE SCHOOL LEVEL

Objective:	**Describes community efforts to prevent and control disease.**
Level:	Grade 8
Title:	*Hectic About Septic*
Vocabulary:	Septic, leaching, hepatitis, typhoid fever
Content	
Generalization:	Clean water is essential for life. In many communities, septic tank treatment of household waste water is used to purify the water. Human wastes are a source of serious threats to health, containing germs that cause forms of hepatitis and typhoid fever. However, when homeowners and communities abide by clean water regulations, these diseases can be prevented.
Materials:	Invitation to a guest speaker from the local sewer utility or public works department.
Initiation:	Invite guest into the classroom to explain the processes household waste water must undergo before it is released into waterways.
Activity:	Give the students the following problem: Local fishermen complain to the local health department that Clean Stream has dead fish floating in it. Technicians from the health department visit the stream and take water samples. Laboratory studies indicate the presence of human waste in the stream. Divide the class into three groups: 1) health department officials, 2) fishermen, and 3) homeowners who own the leaking septic tanks. The students plan a role-play situation. Health department officials try to take action against the homeowners and convince them to repair the damaged tanks. The fishermen expect the homeowners to pay for the lost fishing privileges. The homeowners want to know what they have to do and who is responsible to pay for the repairs and environmental damage. Students are to contact the local health department or sewer utility to determine which state regulations cover the maintenance of community septic tanks. They will need to determine who pays for the repairs and damage to the environment. After they have explored the legal and environmental issues, the students act out their roles.
Closure:	Ask students, "Why do some people choose not to accept responsibility for creating serious health risks like the leaky septic tanks?"

COMMUNITY HEALTH
MIDDLE SCHOOL LEVEL

Objective:	**Concludes that individual participation is essential if community health activities are to be successful.**
Level:	Grade 8
Title:	*Benefits of Health*
Integration:	Social studies, interpersonal
Content	
Generalization:	Most larger communities have health agencies that educate the public about various disorders and provide other services. Many of these agencies rely on volunteer help and donations to operate.
Materials:	List of community health agencies and organizations from text (Fig. 19-7, p. 483)
	Letter to parents explaining the nature of the activity. **Obtain parental approval for this activity.**
Initiation:	Ask students if they or their parents volunteer time or donate money to help health agencies, such as the American Red Cross, American Heart Association, American Cancer Society, or Arthritis Foundation.
Activity:	Students choose one organization from the list of community health agencies and organizations and contact the agency. Students are to ask a representative of the agency if they can use the volunteer help of an eighth grader. If they can use their help, the student is to spend at least 1 hour performing volunteer work for the agency. The work may include canvassing a neighborhood to collect donations, answering the phones, or mailing educational materials. Students are to write a brief synopsis of their experience.
Closure:	Ask, "What roles can individuals play to help health agencies meet their goals?

TEACHING RESOURCES AND STUDENT HANDOUTS

Fig. 1-1
Handout

Brian, the Worm Collector

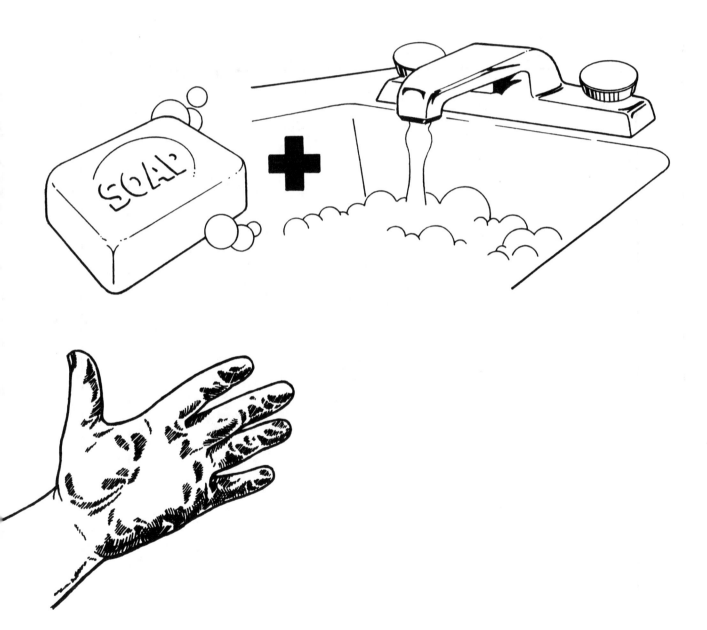

Fig. 1-2
Handout

I am Healthy Because...

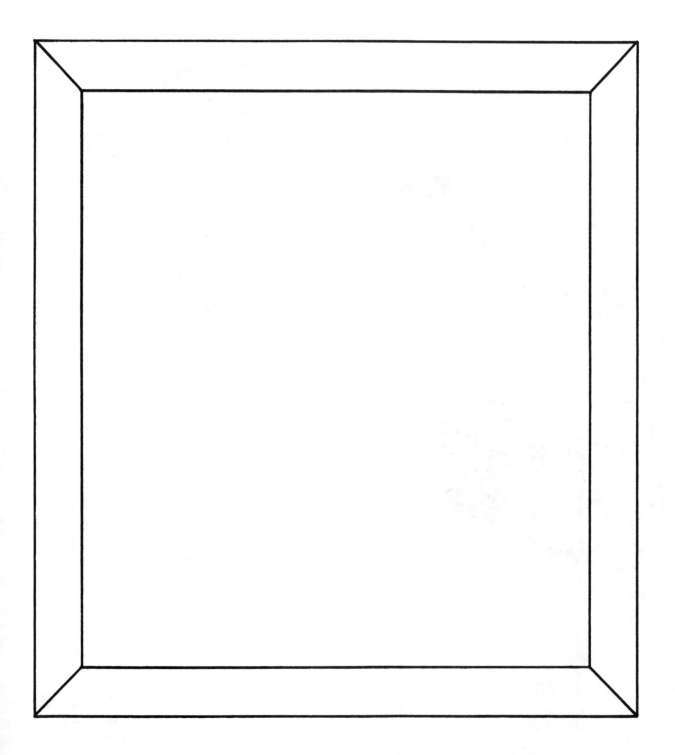

Fig. 1-3
Teacher Resource

Tooth Diagram Poster

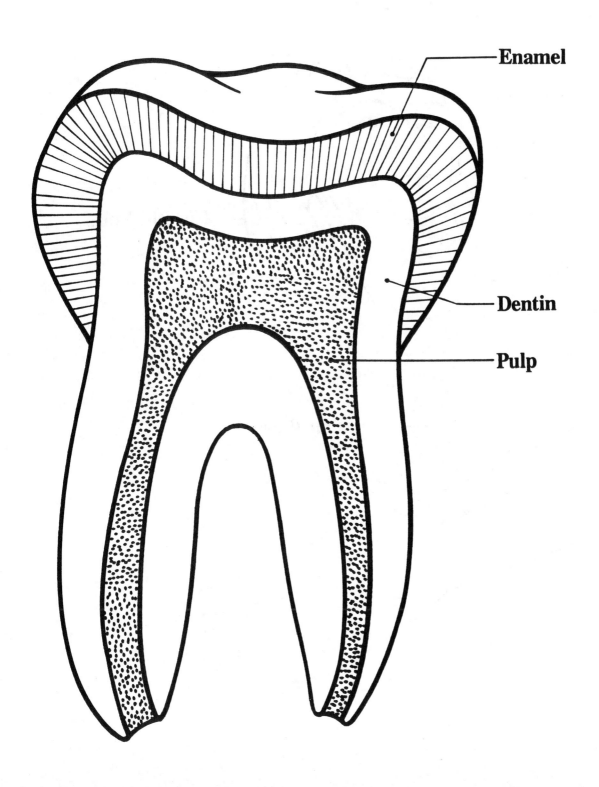

Enamel

Dentin

Pulp

Fig. 1-4
Handout

Locating Your Pulse

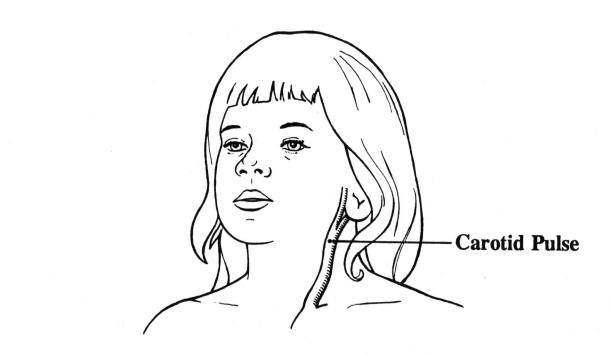

Carotid Pulse

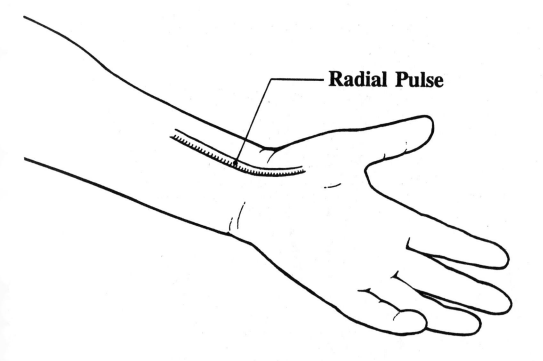

Radial Pulse

Fig. 1-5
Handout

Activities and Calories Burned Chart
   To determine the number of Calories burned while engaged in 1 hour of an activity, find the activity, then multiply the number of Calories burned times your weight in pounds.

Activity	Calories Burned	Activity	Calories Burned
Basketball	3.78	Judo	5.34
Baseball	1.89	Marching	3.84
Climbing hills	3.30	Playing music (sitting)	1.08
Cleaning	1.62	Running, cross-country	4.44
Cooking	1.20	Sewing	0.60
Cycling		Sitting	0.66
5.5 mph	1.74	Skiing, cross-country	4.44
9.4	2.70	Skating	2.28
Racing	4.62	Sleeping	0.54
Eating	0.60	Soccer	3.54
Football	3.60	Standing	0.93
Mowing lawn	3.06	Swimming	
Gymnastics	1.80	Backstroke	4.62
Hiking	2.52	Breaststroke	4.44
Horseback riding		Fast crawl	4.26
Gallop	3.72	Table tennis	1.86
Trotting	3.00	Volleyball	1.32
Ice hockey	5.70	Normal walking pace	2.16
Jogging	4.14	Weight training	1.89
		Wrestling	5.10
		Writing	0.78

Fig. 1-6
Handout

ACTIVITY GRAPH HANDOUT

Name_____

Activity Time Spent/Day

	Mon	Tue	Wed	Thurs	Fri	Sat	Sun
Week 1 Activity Record							
Week 2 Activity Record							
Week 3 Activity Record							
Week 4 Activity Record							
Week 5 Activity Record							
Week 6 Activity Record							
Week 7 Activity Record							
Week 8 Activity Record							

Beginning Skinfolds _____
Ending Skinfolds _____

Fig. 2-1
Handout

Sad Day	Happy Day

Fig. 2-2
Handout

Mentalmeter

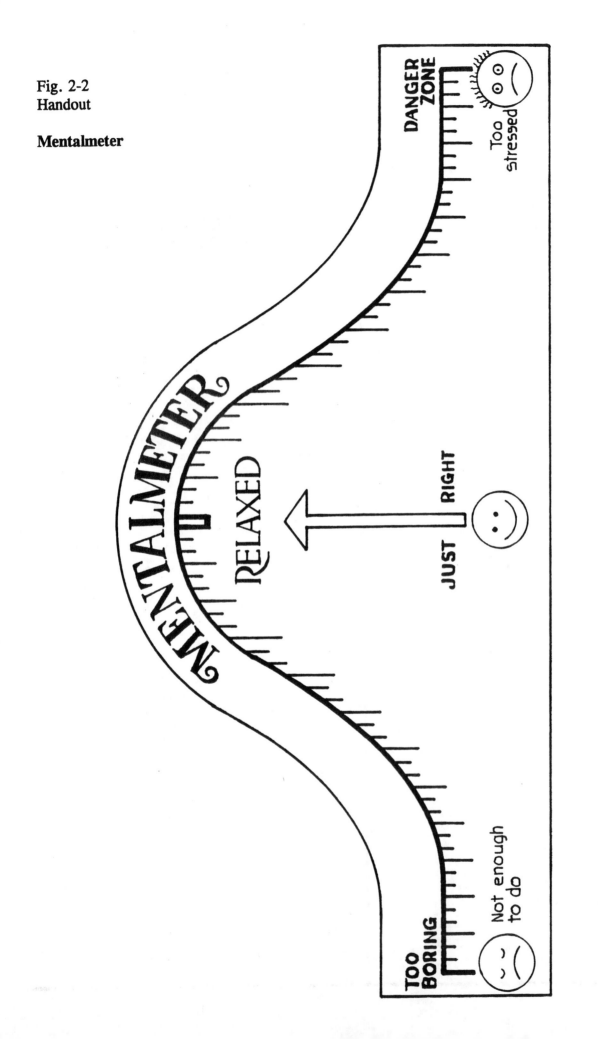

Fig. 2-3
Handout

Peer Power

Role Play 1 (two boys)
    Marcus: Hey, Andre, wanna smoke this joint?
    Andre: Well, I don't know...

(Continue the situation by making up the rest of the action.)

Role Play 2 (two girls) Telephone conversation
    Vanessa: Hi Megan! Let's go rollerblading at the park.
    Megan: I think I'd rather watch TV this afternoon. My mom
            bought a huge bag of chips. Why don't you come over
            and share it with me?

(Continue the situation in which Vanessa and Megan are deciding what to
do with their afternoon.)

Role Play 3 (a girl and boy)   On the couch

    Christy: Matt, you are such a hunk!
    Matt: Thanks, Christy. I think we better work on this
          assignment. It's due tomorrow.
    Christy: Oh, Matt. That stupid project can wait. You know I've
          liked you since the fifth grade. I just want to kiss you!
    Matt: Christy! Your parents are upstairs!

(Continue the situation in which Christy is pressuring Matt for a kiss.)

Fig. 3-1
Teacher Resource

OUR FAMILY TREE BULLETIN BOARD

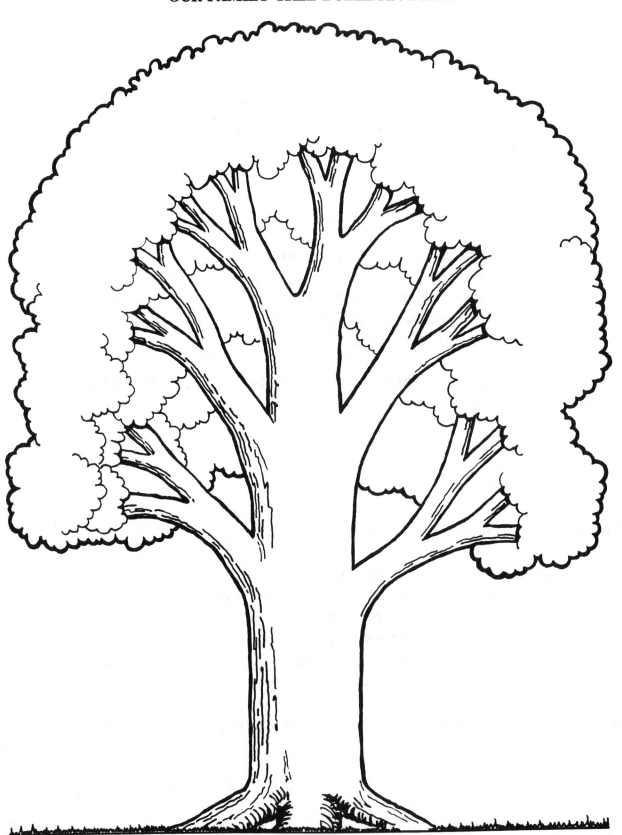

Fig. 3-2
Teacher Resource

CHORE CHART

Student Name	Clean Erasers	Water Plants	Feed Fish	Feed Gerbils	Stack Chairs	Empty Recycle Box	Message Runner	Library Return		

Fig. 3-3
Teacher Resource

Male and Female Body Patterns

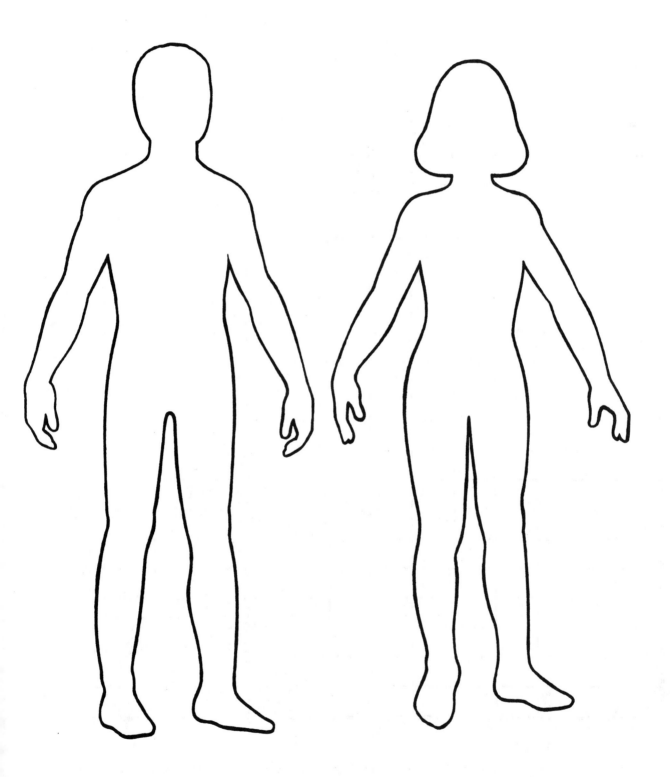

Fig. 4-1
Teacher Resource

Food Pyramid Puzzle

Cut on heavy lines to make the puzzle.

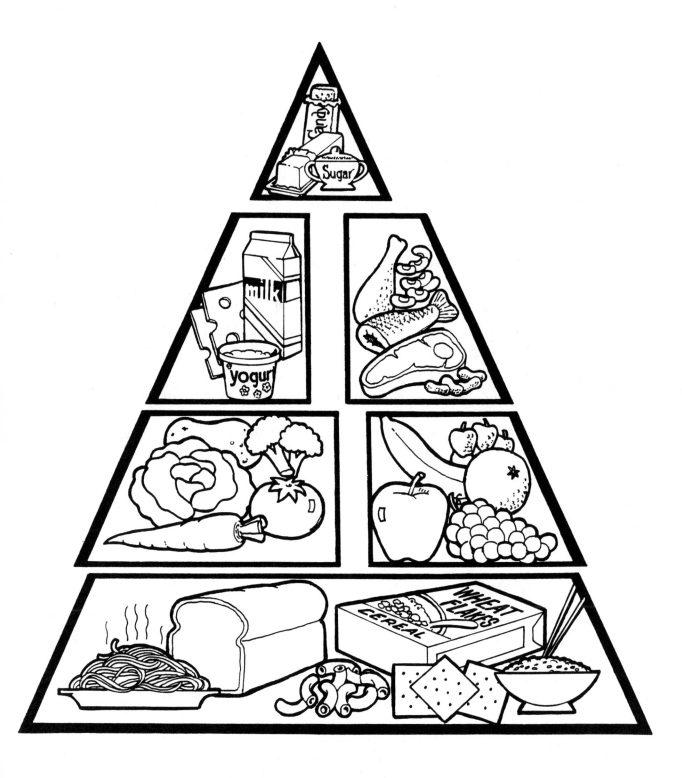

Fig. 4-2
Teacher Resource

FOODGO

Fruits	Vegetables	Meat and Meat Alternates	Milk	Cereals
		Salty snacks and sweets space		

1. Make five different versions of the gameboard using heavy cardboard. Laminate.

2. Make "chips" using heavy cardboard, laminate. Make 28 of each kind of chip.

3. Divide chips into four sets of 84 chips.

4. Place each set of chips in an envelope.

Chips: cut on solid lines.

FAT	PROTEIN	WATER	MINERAL SODIUM	MINERAL CALCIUM	MINERAL IRON
CARBO-HYDRATE	VITAMIN C	VITAMIN A	VITAMIN D	B-VITAMIN B_{12}	FIBER

Fig. 4-2
Teacher Resource

FoodGo Instructions (con't)

Nutrient Function Game Cards: Make out of heavy cardboard. Cut along lines to make cards. Laminate.

Mineral for making hemoglobin in red blood cells (iron)	Vitamin for healthy blood vessels (Vitamin C)
Vitamin for vision (calcium)	Vitamin for strong bones (Vitamin D)
Mineral for making bones (calcium)	Roughage for healthy digestive tract (fiber)
Mineral for making teeth (calcium)	Nutrient for transporting materials in blood (water)
Vitamin for healthy skin (Vitamin A)	Major energy storage (fat)
Mineral for nerve function (calcium)	Building, repairing all cells (protein)
Vitamin for blood (Vitamin B_{12})	Mineral for water balance (sodium)
Energy nutrient (Carbohydrates, protein, or fats)	Energy nutrient (Carbohydrates, protein, or fats)

Fig. 4-3
Handout

A Day in the Life of Joe and Wes

Estimate the amount of Calories each boy expended in 1 day's physical activities. Use the Activities and Calories Burned handout to determine the Calories. Each boy weighs 100 pounds.

Joe's Day

Activity	Time	x Activity Calories	x Body Weight	= Calories Burned
Sleeping	10 hours	x _____	x _____	= _____
Sitting in class	7 hours	x _____	x _____	= _____
Basketball	0.5 hour	x _____	x _____	= _____
Jogging	0.5 hour	x _____	x _____	= _____
Eating	1 hour	x _____	x _____	= _____
Watching TV	2 hours	x _____	x _____	= _____
Playing piano	0.5 hour	x _____	x _____	= _____
Homework	2 hours	x _____	x _____	= _____
Standing	1.5 hours	x _____	x _____	= _____
			Total	_____

Wes's Day

Activity	Time	x Activity Calories	x Body Weight	= Calories Burned
Sleeping	8 hours	x ___	x ___	= ___
Sitting in class	7 hours	x ___	x ___	= ___
Jogging	1.5 hours	x ___	x ___	= ___
Cooking	0.5 hour	x ___	x ___	= ___
Watching TV	2 hours	x ___	x ___	= ___
Homework	2 hours	x ___	x ___	= ___
Eating	1.5 hours	x ___	x ___	= ___
Standing	1 hour	x ___	x ___	= ___
			Total	___

QUESTIONS:

1. Which boy needs more Calories? _____

2. For each boy, which activity expended the most Calories?
   Joe _____   Wes _____

3. For each boy, which activity expended the least Calories?
   Joe _____   Wes _____

Fig. 4-4
Teacher Resource

Key to: A Day in the Life of Joe and Wes

Estimate the amount of Calories each boy expended in 1 day's physical
activities. Use the Activities and Calories Burned handout to determine the Calories.
Each boy weighs 100 pounds.

Joe's Day

Activity	Time	x Activity Calories	x Body Weight	= Calories Burned
Sleeping	10 hours	x 0.54	x 100	= 540
Sitting in class	7 hours	x 0.66	x 100	= 462
Basketball	0.5 hour	x 3.78	x 100	= 189
Jogging	0.5 hour	x 4.14	x 100	= 207
Eating	1 hour	x 0.60	x 100	= 60
Watching TV	2 hours	x 0.66 (sitting)	x 100	= 132
Playing piano	0.5 hour	x 1.08	x 100	= 54
Homework	2 hours	x 0.66 (sitting)	x 100	= 132
Standing	1.5 hours	x 0.93	x 100	= 140
			Total	1916 Calories

Wes's Day

Activity	Time	x Activity Calories	x Body Weight	= Calories Burned
Sleeping	8 hours	x 0.54	x 100	= 459
Sitting in class	7 hours	x 0.66	x 100	= 462
Jogging	1.5 hours	x 4.14	x 100	= 621
Cooking	0.5 hour	x 1.20	x 100	= 60
Watching TV	2 hours	x 0.66	x 100	= 132
Homework	2 hours	x 0.66(sitting)	x 100	= 132
Eating	1.5 hours	x 0.60	x 100	= 90
Standing	1 hour	x 0.93	x 100	= 93
			Total	2049 Calories

QUESTIONS:
1. Which boy needs more Calories? Wes

2. For each boy, which activity expended the most Calories?
   Joe Sleeping   Wes Jogging

3. For each boy, which activity expended the least Calories?
   Joe Playing piano   Wes Cooking

Fig. 4-5
Handout

Menu Guide
   Breakfast: _____
              _____
              _____
              _____

   Snack: _____
          _____

   Lunch: _____
          _____
          _____
          _____
          _____

   Snack: _____
          _____

   Dinner: _____
           _____
           _____
           _____
           _____

   Snack: _____
          _____

Fig. 4-6
Handout

A Week's Worth of Differences

Kyle has been maintaining his weight for several weeks. According to his doctor, he needs about 2300 Calories each day. He decided to keep track of his caloric intakes and expenditures to see why he has not been able to gain any weight. Determine the difference between his caloric intake and the recommended level of Calories for his age group (2300 Calories) for each day. If he has eaten more than 2300 Calories, calculate the difference and write a + sign in front of the amount of Calories. If he has not consumed enough Calories to meet the 2300 level, write the difference and place a - sign in front of the amount of Calories.

Monday
Total Calories eaten: 2000
Needs: 2300
Difference:

Tuesday
Total Calories eaten: 1500
Needs: 2300
Difference:

Wednesday
Total Calories eaten: 2500
Needs: 2300
Difference:

Thursday
Total Calories eaten: 2000
Needs: 2300
Difference:

Friday
Total Calories eaten: 3000
Needs: 2300
Difference:

Saturday
Total Calories eaten: 2300
Needs: 2300
Difference:

Sunday
Total Calories eaten: 2400
Needs: 2300
Difference:

1. Calculate the total excess or deficit of Calories for the 7 days.

2. A pound of body fat represents 3500 Calories of stored energy. Will Kyle lose or gain a pound by the end of this week? Explain.

Fig. 4-7
Teacher Resource

Key for: A Week's Worth of Differences

   Kyle has been maintaining his weight for several weeks. According to his doctor, he need about 2300 Calories each day. He decided to keep track of his caloric intakes and expenditur to see why he has not been able to gain any weight. Determine the difference between his caloric intake and the recommended level of Calories for his age group (2300 Calories) for ea day. If he has eaten more than 2300 Calories, calculate the difference and write a + sign in front of the amount of Calories. If he has not consumed enough Calories to meet the 2300 level, write the difference and place a - sign in front of the amount of Calories.

Monday		**Tuesday**		**Wednesday**	
Total Calories eaten:	2000	Total Calories eaten:	1500	Total Calories eaten:	2500
Needs:	2300	Needs:	2300	Needs:	2300
Difference:	- 300	Difference:	- 800	Difference:	+ 200

Thursday		**Friday**		**Saturday**	
Total Calories eaten:	2000	Total Calories eaten:	3000	Total Calories eaten:	2300
Needs:	2300	Needs:	2300	Needs:	2300
Difference:	- 300	Difference:	+ 700	Difference:	0

Sunday	
Total Calories eaten:	2400
Needs:	2300
Difference:	+ 100

1. Calculate the total excess or deficit of Calories for the 7 days.

2. A pound of body fat represents 3500 Calories of stored energy. Will Kyle lose or gain a pound by the end of this week? Explain.
   Kyle will not lose or gain a pound because he has a deficit of 400 Calories for the week To lose a pound he would have to have a 3500 Calorie deficit. To gain a pound, he woul need to have an excess of 3500 Calories.

Fig. 4-8
Handout

Marta's Latest Weight Loss Diet

Marta read about this diet plan in one of her mother's magazines.

Analyze the plan using the Food Pyramid, and decide if this plan has the characteristics of a reasonable weight loss program.
1. Does it contain familiar foods from all food groups?
2. Does it include any promises or gimmicks?
3. Does it limit Calories to less than 1200 per day?
4. Does it include a physical activity program?
5. Can one follow this plan for a lifetime?

<u>Diet Plan</u>

Breakfast:	Water, tea, coffee, or diet soda
Lunch:	Mixed salad with low-fat dressing
	Plain roll
	Diet soda
Snack:	Diet Soda and LOSEIT wafer (100 Calories)
Dinner:	One envelope of LOSEIT powder mixed with 8 oz. of skim milk
	LOSEIT Label:
	Calories per serving when mixed with 8 oz. skim milk = 300
	Contains 100% of a day's recommended vitamins
Snack:	LOSEIT wafer (100 Calories)

LOSEIT ADVERTISEMENT and package instructions:

Before starting the LOSEIT weight loss plan, check with your doctor. The LOSEIT plan has been used by millions of satisfied people to lose weight and keep it off without starving or exercising. We guarantee that you will lose weight fast on this plan! Fat just melts off your body. Just follow the plan every day, and in 1 week lose up to 10 pounds! That's up to 3 inches off of your thighs, 6 inches off of your hips, and 3 inches off of your waist. MEN love LOSEIT too! Easily removes that "spare tire" without back-breaking sit-ups! SAFE and EFFECTIVE! USE IT AND LOSE IT with LOSEIT!

1. Analyze this diet plan and its claims. Should you follow this diet plan to lose weight? Explain.

Fig. 4-9
Teacher Resource

Key to: Marta's Latest Weight Loss Diet
Marta read about this diet plan in one of her mother's magazines.

Analyze the plan using the Food Pyramid, and decide if this plan has the characteristics of a reasonable weight loss program.
1. Does it contain familiar foods from all food groups?
2. Does it include any promises or gimmicks?
3. Does it limit Calories to less than 1200 per day?
4. Does it include a physical activity program?
5. Can one follow this plan for a lifetime?

	Diet Plan
Breakfast:	Water, tea, coffee, or diet soda
Lunch:	Mixed salad with low-fat dressing
	Plain roll
	Diet soda
Snack:	Diet Soda and LOSEIT wafer (100 Calories)
Dinner:	One envelope of LOSEIT powder mixed with 8 oz. of skim milk
	LOSEIT Label:
	Calories per serving when mixed with 8 oz. skim milk = 300
	Contains 100% of a day's recommended vitamins
Snack:	LOSEIT wafer (100 Calories)

LOSEIT ADVERTISEMENT and package instructions:

Before starting the LOSEIT weight loss plan, check with your doctor. The LOSEIT plan has been used by millions of satisfied people to lose weight and keep it off with out starving or exercising. We guarantee that you will lose weight fast on this plan! Fat just melts off your body. Just follow the plan every day, and in 1 week lose up to 10 pounds! That's up to 3 inches off of your thighs, 6 inches off of your hips, and 3 inches off of your waist. MEN love LOSEIT too! Easily removes that "spare tire" without back-breaking sit-ups! SAFE and EFFECTIVE! USE IT AND LOSE IT with LOSEIT!

1. Analyze this diet plan and its claims. Should you follow this diet plan to lose weight? Explain.
    This diet plan does not meet the recommended amounts of foods from all food groups of the Food Pyramid. It is too low in Calories, and it does not recommend any increase in physical activity. Furthermore, it uses a synthetic food product that contains 100% of certain vitamins, but no mention of protein, minerals, or fiber content is given. The guarantee is meaningless. A person will lose weight on this very low-calorie plan, but with these kinds of diets, the lost weight is regained rapidly when the person returns to their usual eating patterns. One cannot follow this kind of diet for a lifetime without becoming very bored with the plan or experiencing health problems.

Fig. 5-1
Handout

When I am Sick...

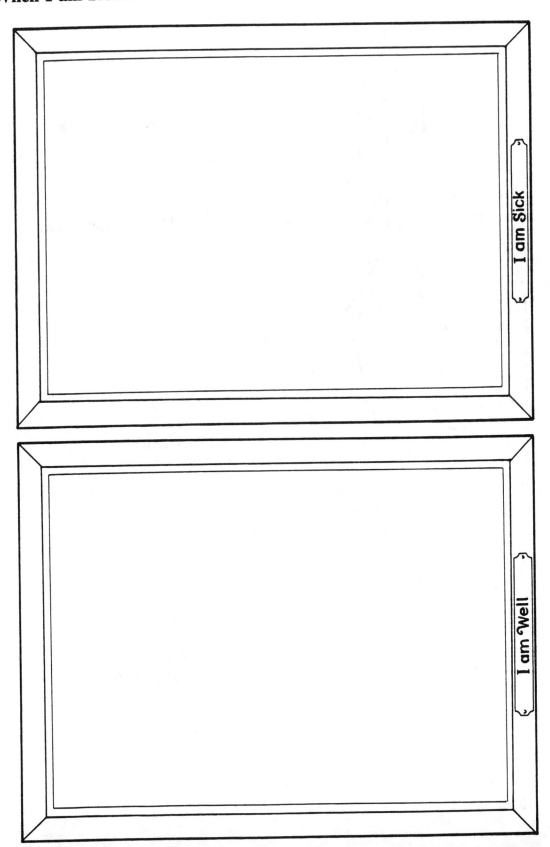

Fig. 6-1
Teacher Resource

Instruction for Bottle Lung Chamber

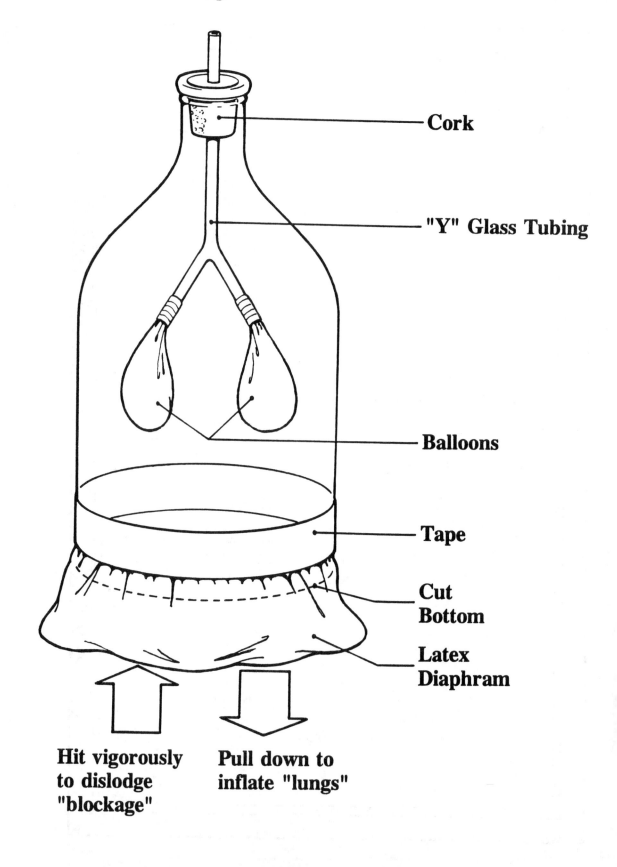

Cork

"Y" Glass Tubing

Balloons

Tape

Cut Bottom

Latex Diaphram

Hit vigorously to dislodge "blockage"

Pull down to inflate "lungs"

Fig. 7-1
Handout

Health-Care Products At My House

Student Name_____

Name of health-care product _____
Made by _____

Ask your parents:

1. Where was the product purchased? _____

2. Price of the product_____

3. Why was the product purchased? _____
   _____
   _____
   _____

4. How necessary is this product? _____ very   ____somewhat   ____ not very

5. How long have you been using this particular product? _____

6. What do you like about this product _____
   _____

7. Do you buy similar products from other companies or only this particular brand name?

   _____ similar products from other companies   _____ only this brand name

8. If you only buy this particular product, why? _____
   _____

9. What would make you decide to try a similar product from another company?
   _____
   _____
   _____

Fig. 7-2
Teacher Resource

Health Worker ID Cards
Copy these cards on plain heavy cardboard and laminate.

DOCTOR	RESTAURANT INSPECTOR
NURSE	FIREMAN
PHARMACIST	POLICEMAN
DENTIST	DENTAL HYGIENIST

lth Care Product Cards
y these cards on plain heavy cardboard and laminate.

TOOTHPASTE	ANTI-ITCH CREAM
DENTAL FLOSS	ANTI-BACTERIAL CREAM
SHAMPOO	HEADACHE PILLS
SOAP	STOMACH MEDICINE HYGIENIST

Fig. 7-4
Handout

Looking at Labels

Student Name_____

Name of product: _____

Weight of entire package: _____

Price: _____

List of ingredients:

Questions:

1. This product contains more _____ than any other ingredient.

2. Which ingredient is in the smallest amount? _____

3. Explain how you can use this information to be a better shopper.

Fig. 7-5
Handout

Label Fables

Student Name _____

Food Product A

Product name _____

Serving size _____

Servings / container _____

Number of Calories / serving ____

Total Calories in container ____

(**Hint**: The number of servings in container x   number of Calories / serving = total Calories in container)

Number of Calories from fat _____

% of Calories from fat ____

Food Product B

Product name _____

Serving size _____

Servings / container _____

Number of Calories / serving ____

Total Calories in container ____

Number of Calories from fat ____

% of Calories from fat ____

(**Hint**: Take the number of Calories from fat, and divide that number by the total number of Calories. You will have a decimal. Take the decimal and multiply it times 100 to get the percent of Calories from fat.)

Foods with less than 30% of their Calories from fat are considered to be healthier than those with higher fat percentages.

Was either of your food products less than 30% fat? ___yes   ___ no

If yes, which one? _____

Fig. 7-6
Handout

Brand Name vs. Generic

Student Name _____

Compare two similar health-care products: one an advertised, brand name product; the other, a generic type.

Brand Name Product	Generic Product
Name of product _____	Name of product _____
Price _____	Price _____
Weight of product _____ounces	Weight of product _____ ounces
Price /ounce _____	Price / ounce _____
List of ingredients:	List of ingredients:

Label:
Colors used: _____   Colors used: _____
             _____   _____

How attractive is the design?

_____   _____

Claims:

Does the manufacturer make any claims about the effectiveness of the product?
_____yes _____ no   _____ yes _____no

If yes, describe the claims:

Which product would you select? Explain why you would select it.

Fig. 7-7
Handout

Aisle Appeal

Student Name _____

Name of Store _____

Cereals:

How many shelves are used on one side of an aisle to stack cereal products? _____

List three brand names of cereals on the highest shelf:
a.
b.
c.

List three brand names of cereals on the middle shelves:
a.
b.
c.

List three brand names of cereals on the bottom shelf:
a.
b.
c.

Which shelves have the most cereals that are marketed to young children?
_____ top   _____ middle   _____ bottom

Which shelves have the most cereals that are marketed to older adults?
___top   ___ middle   ___ bottom

Which shelves have the least expensive brands of cereals?
___ top   ___ middle   ___ bottom

Which brands of cereals have the most attractive packaging?

_____

_____

What makes the package so attractive?

Does the attractiveness of the cereal package have anything to do with its cost?

Do you think cereals are shelved from top to bottom for any marketing reasons?

Fig. 7-8
Handout

Comic Appeal

Student Name _____

Find the vitamin/mineral pill section of a pharmacy, grocery, or variety store. Answer the following questions about the nutrient pills.

1. Name of store_____

2. Number of shelves with vitamin/mineral supplements _____

3. Where are these products located in the store?_____

    _____

    _____

4. How many brands of the following nutrients do they offer?

    Vitamin C _____

    Vitamin E _____

    Beta carotene _____

    Iron _____

    Calcium _____

5. How many brands of children's vitamin/ mineral pills are on the shelves? _____

6. How are the labels for children's nutrient pills different from those used for adult pills?

Fig. 7-9
Handout

Ad Fads   Student Name _____

Look through magazines you or your parents receive. Locate an advertisement for a tobacco or alcoholic beverage product. Answer the following questions about the ad.

1. Name of the tobacco or alcoholic beverage featured in the ad_____

2. What do you like about the ad? _____

_____

3. What do you <u>dislike</u> about the ad? _____

_____

_____

4. The ad's message indicates that people who use the product:

are attractive   _____yes

have money   _____ yes

are successful   _____ yes

are happy   _____ yes

are healthy   _____ yes

have friends   _____ yes

(describe any other characteristics) _____

5. On the basis of this ad, would you use this product?   ___ yes   ___no

Explain.

Fig. 7-10
Handout

Designing a Study

Invent a health anecdote or a person's testimonial about a health product. For example, people who use aloe on burns say it leaves no scar. Or, eating fish makes you smarter. Write this as a question that could be researched. Using the example of aloe, the question could be, "What is the usefulness of aloe in preventing burns from scarring?"
Design a scientific study to test this question by following the steps listed below:

1. Choose your subjects. Will you test your question on animal or human subject? How many subjects will you need?

2. Divide your subjects into a control group and an experimental group. Explain what will happen to each subject in the control and experimental groups.

3. How long will your study take?

4. Conduct your study and gather results. You may find no effect, some degree of benefit, or possibly some degree of harm from your treatment.

5. Write a brief discussion of your results. What do they mean? What kinds of future studies can be conducted to examine different aspects of your original question?

Fig. 7-11
Handout

The Claim Game

Student Name _____

Read each of the following advertising claims. Analyze each for being a misleading statement. The following questions will help you determine if the statements are misleading:

1. Is the claim difficult to prove?

2. Does the claim use personal testimonials to support it?

3. What evidence is given to support the claim?

4. Could other advertisers make the same claim?

5. Are "fad" words used in the claim or on the label?

6. Does current scientific knowledge fail to support the claim?

Examples:
Check out the following claims:

a. "Nine out of ten doctors agree..."

b. "Guaranteed to melt pounds off your body ..."

c. "Rich in antioxidants..."

d. "Proven after 25 years of scientific research..."

e. "More youthful appearance..."

f. "Makes wrinkles disappear..."

g. "Twenty-five percent more energy..."

Fig. 7-12
Handout

Choosing a Health Advisor

Student Name _____

Name of the person being interviewed _____

What is their relationship to the student? _____

1. Ask the person to identify a favorite health advisor (doctor, dentist, etc.).

   Type of health advisor_____

2. Ask, "Why do you like this health advisor?

3. Ask the person to identify a type of health advisor whom they do not like.

   Type of health advisor _____

4. Ask, "Why don't you like this type of health advisor?"

5. Ask, "What are the characteristics of a good health advisor?"

Fig. 8-1
Handout

Pros and Cons   Student Names _____

                                     _____

Read the following situation, determine the alternative choices, and list the **pros** and **cons** for each alternative.

Example: Laura does not want to go to school because of a scheduled spelling test. Before breakfast, she tells her mother that her stomach is upset. Her mother takes her temperature and says, "You don't have a fever. I think you can go to school. Don't you have a spelling test today?"

   What should Laura tell her mother? What should she do? What are her choices? List the **pros** and **cons** of Laura's decision to stay home from school.

Situation: While walking home from school, Ben and Jason see Cory, Jason's older brother, hanging around the high school with a couple of older boys whom they do not recognize. "Hey, Jason," calls Cory, "Come over here." As the boys approach, they smell a strange odor. It doesn't smell like cigarettes. "Try smoking this." One of the unknown boys offers Jason a rolled-up piece of paper with something that looks like oregano inside. What are Jason's choices? What are the **pros** and **cons** of each of those choices?

   One of the other boys is drinking from a beer bottle hidden in a paper bag. "Want some of this?" he says, while offering the bottle to Ben. What are Ben's choices? What are the **pros** and **cons** of each of those choices?

Fig. 9-1
Handout

Find the Pollutant

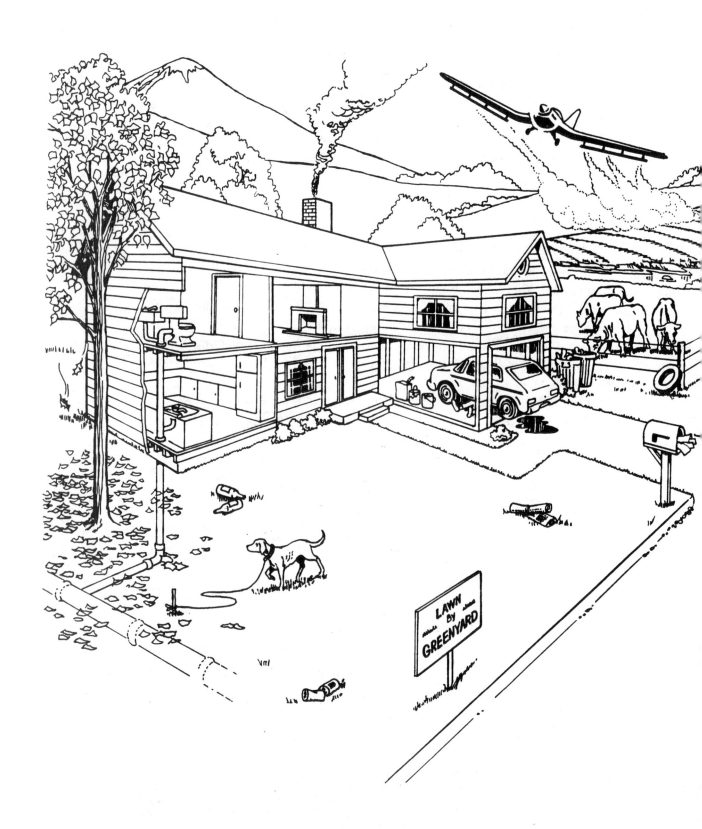

Fig. 9-2
Teacher Resource

Key to: Find The Pollutant

Sources of Pollution:
    Bathroom wastewater
    Kitchen wastewater
    Fireplace smoke
    Lead paint chips
    Aesbestos used in old shingles or for insulation
    Yard waste (leaf and grass clippings that are not composted)
    Pesticides applied to yard
    Fertilizers on field (these can run-off into streams)
    Farm animals (wastes can run-off into streams)
    Car
    Trash
    Newsprint
    "Junk mail"
    Paint cans with paint remaining
    Tire
    Dog (wastes can runn-off into streams)
    Can (aluminum can be recycled)
    Bottle (glass can be recycled)

Fig. 9-3
Teacher Resource

Plastic Milk Carton Bird Feeder Instructions

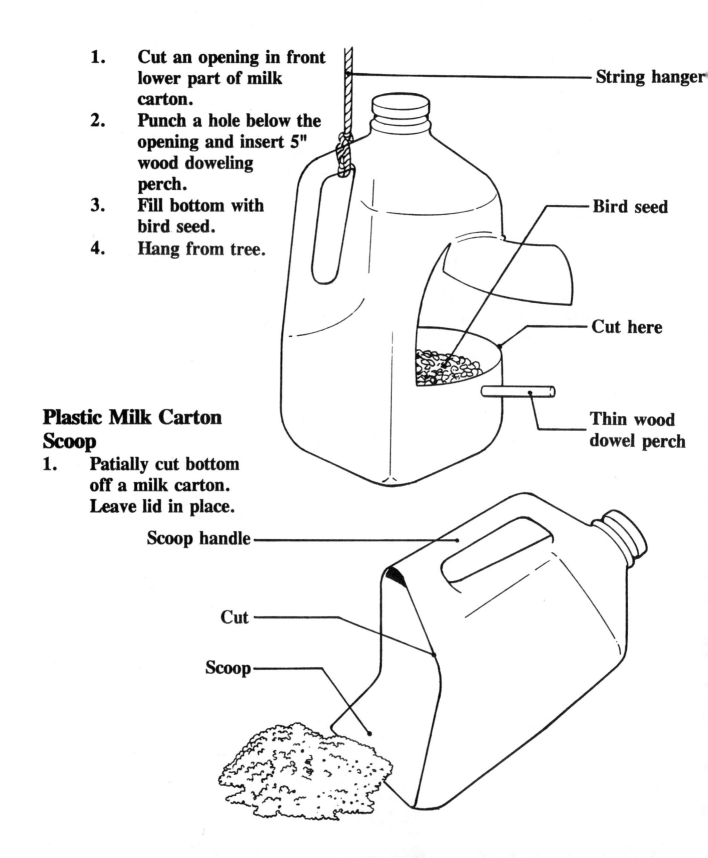

1. Cut an opening in front lower part of milk carton.
2. Punch a hole below the opening and insert 5" wood doweling perch.
3. Fill bottom with bird seed.
4. Hang from tree.

String hanger

Bird seed

Cut here

Thin wood dowel perch

Plastic Milk Carton Scoop

1. Patially cut bottom off a milk carton. Leave lid in place.

Scoop handle

Cut

Scoop

Fig. 10-1
Handout

Match the drawing with the Health Helper

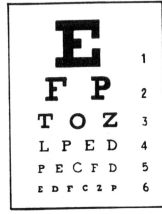

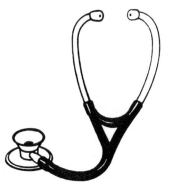

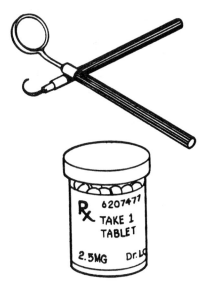

Dentist

Pharmacist

Doctor

Eye Doctor